Because cowards get
cancer too...

C

Because cowards get
cancer too...

John Diamond

VERMILION
LONDON

To Nigella

11 12 13 14 15 16 17 18 19 20

First published in 1998 in Great Britain by Vermilion,
an imprint of Ebury Press, Random House,
20 Vauxhall Bridge Road, London SW1V 2SA

Paperback edition published in 1999

Random House Australia (Pty) Limited
20 Alfred Street, Milsons Point, Sydney,
New South Wales 2061, Australia

Random House New Zealand Limited
18 Poland Road, Glenfield,
Auckland 10, New Zealand

Random House South Africa (Pty) Limited
Endulini, 5a Jubilee Road,
Parktown 2193, South Africa

Random House UK Limited Reg. No. 954009

Papers used by Vermilion are natural, recyclable products made from wood
grown in sustainable forests.

Printed by Bookmarque Ltd, Croydon, Surrey

A CIP catalogue record for this book
is available from the British Library

ISBN 0-09-181665-3

'There are journeys none of us wish to take. But sometimes we must. John Diamond is the exquisite cartographer of a savage landscape. C, which will become a classic, is not only about the cruelty of cancer. It is about life as it is, arbitrary, brutal and glorious. Read it with gratitude.'

Josephine Hart

'Funny, honest and inspirational.'

GQ Active

'His many admirers will buy this book because the "old", wry Diamond speaks in every taut phrase. Anyone unfamiliar with the story should buy it because they will be gripped as if by a thriller, by a narrative which also teaches much about medicine and mortality.'

Bel Mooney, The Times

In 20 years' time, if – touch wood, please God, all of that malarkey – I am still around, how will I feel about a bad back? I mean, a *really* bad back – the sort of ricked back I had a few years ago when I thought a kidney had burst and I couldn't move for a couple of days, and announced that things couldn't possibly get worse than this, and that this was the greatest medical indignity a man could suffer.

Or a cold – how will I feel about one of those colds when you can't breathe, or think, or write or imagine what it was like before the onset of the cold? Will I still feel about those everyday reasons for giving up as I did before 27 March 1997?

That was the date I was diagnosed as having cancer. In statistical terms that's no big deal: some hundreds of thousands of Britons get the same diagnosis every year. In fact many of them get a rather scarier diagnosis than I did, for although my odds changed over the year, at first I was given a 92 per cent chance of a full cure. Mine was just a small local cancer, they said, and one that could be scared off with a little radiotherapy. It wasn't, as it turned out, but it didn't matter for nobody receives a diagnosis of even the least invasive cancer with anything but fear and dread.

Over the next year or so the illness took over my life. How could it not? For all that the counsellors beseech cancer patients to carry on as before, it's impossible. Impossible because of the constraints imposed by the illness and the often worse constraints imposed by the cure. Impossible because, however good the prognosis sounds, it can only ever be equivocal and even the best-augured cancers can turn into fatal ones. Tell anyone that you have cancer and what they'll hear is that you're

C

about to die. Why would they not? It's what you heard when you got the diagnosis, after all.

As I write, the odds on my being cured of my own cancer have dropped but I am assured still that I am curable. So let's say I get myself cured, that I go to the hospital one day and they say 'That's it, Mr Diamond. We've checked every one of your cells and not one of them's a cancerous one.' Is that it? Do I go back to being the man I was before, felled by the slightest backache, raging at the first cold of the winter? Or am I a new man with a new perspective, ever conscious that a cold is not cancer, that a bad back is not cancer, that any illness is bearable which doesn't carry the threat of death?

I don't know, nor will I for – fingers crossed, *deo volente*, *inshallah* – 20 years, but my suspicion is that once you've had that diagnosis it stays with you for good. Like a lapsed religion it may not be at the front of your mind all the time but it is yawning away there at the back, just waiting for those moments when it needs to come forward and remind you that you are part of that community which touched death and touches it still, the community which has seen a doctor look at his boots and say 'I'm sorry, but...'

I am, as absolute laymen go, fairly well versed in the language of medicine. As a general journalist coming from a family which includes a retired biochemist and a sometime clinical pharmacologist I have found myself apparently able to write the odd piece about medicine, to present science shows on TV, to write a sceptical medical column in a newspaper. Even before I got the bad news I understood the difference between chemotherapy and radiotherapy and had some basic idea of what a CT scanner did and why it did it.

And yet when the news came through I had no idea where to .

turn. I had some vague notion that there were groups of cancer sufferers who would meet to share stories and give each other solace, and organisations which handed out carefully composed information sheets in Hindi and Greek. I knew that I could sit at a computer screen and sift through a million pages of high-level science and learn the most intimate details of the mating habits of the squamous cell carcinoma.

But none of these would tell me quickly what I needed to know, which was how would cancer affect me – what was it like to be a person with cancer, to deal with the pain and the fear and the anger?

I'm still not sure I do know, nor that I ever will: as in most things I suspect that there is a lot which, at the moment of death, will become apparent and that only then will I say 'So that's what it's like to live with cancer for all those years.'

Meanwhile I have an inkling of an idea about what cancer is, and what it does physically and mentally and about how it's cured. I know more than I once did about what people say to you when you tell them you have cancer, and what they think, and the many mad ways they believe you can be cured. And for some while now I have written about some of these things in my weekly *Times* column, and readers have written to me and said they wished I'd been writing before they heard their own diagnosis, or that of their spouse or their child or their parent or their friend.

This isn't a collection of those columns, although there are a few of them reproduced here, but rather an attempt to write the book I was looking for the night I got the bad news. It isn't a medical textbook, although I've tried to explain something of the science of cancer and its cures, nor is it a book of worthily positive thoughts, although I pass on, for what they're worth,

C

some of the positive thoughts which have occurred to me over the past year or so. If you or yours have received a cancerous diagnosis it probably won't help you get through the nights of fear or the long days of treatment. Or not help you except to tell you that the one thing I learned is that my reaction to the diagnosis and the treatment was nothing like I expected it to be.

There are some other things this book isn't. It isn't a book about a battle against cancer because I despise the set of warlike metaphors that so many apply to cancer. My antipathy to the language of battles and fights has nothing to do with pacifism and everything to do with a hatred for the sort of morality which says that only those who fight hard against their cancer survive it or deserve to survive it – the corollary being that those who lose the fight deserved to do so.

It isn't a book of last gasp cures for cancer. Don't get me wrong: if you find that homoeopathy or the Bach Flower Remedies get you through the long nights then I'm genuinely happy for you. It may even be that if I get too near the edge I might join you at that well of alternative solace. Meanwhile, though, I know that the many advances which have been made against cancer in the past 30 years, and the reason why twice as many sufferers live for five years after diagnosis as was the case 60 years ago, is because the medical orthodoxy, for all its arrogance and self-serving smugness, knows more about the reasons we get cancer and the ways of stopping cancer spreading than the most knowledgeable naturopath.

This book is about my cancer and is, I hope, part of my cure. Or if not that, then part of my reconciliation with the fact that whatever happens I will live with cancer for the rest of my life, and with the understanding that this doesn't mean there aren't still a few good times to come.

I wrote the book as the cancer and its treatment were continuing, although the time-lag varies from chapter to chapter, from event to event. I've tried to even out the effect of this as much as I can, but the fact remains that there are times when I was in some pain while writing about happiness and other times when I was leading an almost normal life and writing about events which scare me still to think of them.

There are people I want to thank. You will, I hope, indulge me to the extent of the single page I need in order to do this. Without some of them I wouldn't be here at all; without others there would have been times when being here wouldn't have been worth the effort.

At the Marsden I want to grasp everyone – cleaners, professors of surgery, the rather distracted Chelsea women who volunteer to work in the outpatients tea shop – with a firm hand and look damply into their eyes. The Marsden really is how hospitals should be run: intelligently, flexibly, always engendering hope. In particular, I want to thank all the nurses on Weston Ward who suffered without demur my temper tantrums, the BBC's cameras and finding themselves unexpectedly the subject of newspaper columns. The doctors who are named in the following chapters already know about my gratitude, but let me offer it again and in particular to Peter Rhŷs Evans, Michael Henk, Nicholas Breach, Cyril Fisher, Snehal Patel, Daniel Archer, Sarah Howells, Peter Williamson, Con Irving and Aina Grieg, Karen Golden, men and women who claim they are just doing their job when they appear, calm and unruffled, like Mills and Boon doctors, on a Sunday evening to explain what's going on, or take calls in the small hours to come and sort my throat out. Many thanks also to my GP, Dr Terence Mulligan.

My friends were, and continue to be, remarkable. In particular

C

Michael Bywater, Ruthie Rogers, Josephine Hart, Chaim Tannenbaum, Roy Greenslade, Gill Morgan, Nick Wapshott, Charles Elton, Lucy Heller, Christine Walker, Alan Yentob, Philippa Walker, Victor Sebestyen and Brian King have given support and succour, asked all the right questions and stopped me believing that being a honking, dribbling fool is necessarily much worse than what I was before the big operation. But I should also rectify an omission from the original text: the most useful of the reference books over the past couple of years has been Dr Robert Buckman's *What You Really Need to Know About Cancer* (Pan Books). Subsequently, Rob has become a cherished friend who I feel I've known for 20 years longer than I have.

At home Cheryl Robinson was no end of help with the children. Lisa Grillo arrived from Italy just before my last operation and has helped make the unbearable less so. Kate Mellor has cheerfully kept my affairs in order since before I knew my affairs needed to be put in order: I owe them all a particular debt of thanks. As I do to my beloved parents, who really shouldn't have had to go through this sort of thing at this stage, and Nigella's family who were supportive above and beyond the call of in-lawly duty.

I should mention my children, Cosima and Bruno, who are two-thirds of my reason for living and, finally, and most of all, Nigella whom I love beyond measure and who kept me alive as much as did any medicine.

John Diamond, London 1998 and 1999

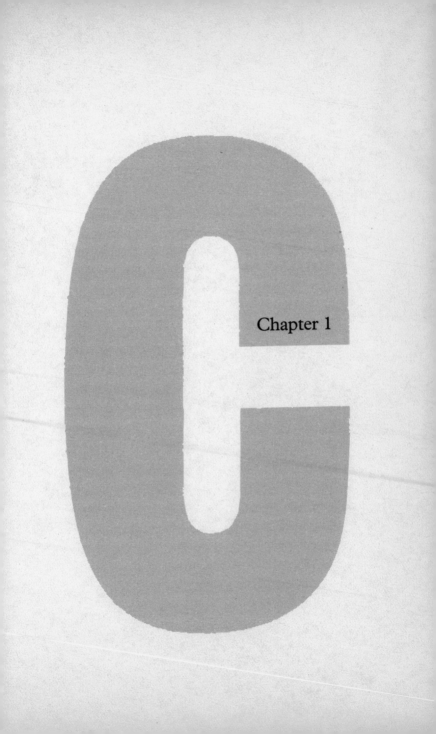

Chapter 1

In the face of such overwhelming statistical possibilities, hypochondria has always seemed to me to be the only rational position to take on life. Consider, by the time you hit 40, your tattered heart has already thumped out a billion and a half beats: what can the chances be of any organ doing anything a billion and a half times and never making a mistake? Your 30 trillion or so cells have each replicated themselves a few thousand times: how could it possibly not be that a few of these cells would band together in that state of cytological anarchy which leads to cancer and death?

Consider anything the body does over and over, asleep and awake, consider the peril it invites every time it gets into a car, breathes a lungful – 150 million times a year, not counting the hours of panicky hyperventilation – of sour and sickly city air, eats something too fatty or not fatty enough, and you are considering impending death.

As it happens it was always the heart attack I was expecting and not just because as a sometime smoking, unexercised and overweight man of fortyish I was drumming my fingers only barely subconsciously while I waited for the smack in the chest to come along; I'd imagined death as something which would give me just enough time to be terrified but not long enough to do anything about it.

But as it turns out it was cancer which got me. Or is, as I write, getting me.

Accidents happen but illness creeps up on you. Only in retrospect do you realise that you'd been ill all along. Of course as a hypochondriac I'd always known that I'd been ill all along, but I'd assumed a symptomless illness which ground me down not with its various discomforts but with its very existence. A hypochondriac friend once told me of a hypochondriac friend of

C

his who told his doctor that he had a fatal disease. 'Really?' said the doctor, 'that's terrible. What are the symptoms?'

'That's the worst thing about it,' said the friend of the friend in absolute seriousness. 'There are none.'

When my friend told me the story we both laughed because we knew we were meant to laugh, but it wasn't genuine laughter. It's impossible to laugh and empathise at the same time.

But just as being paranoid doesn't mean they're not out to get you, so being a hypochondriac doesn't mean you're not about to die.

A year or so ago I had a series of random colds, aches, agues and minor swellings which were sufficiently real to warrant a blood test. It was what we in Britain with our essentially medieval approach to medical taxonomy call glandular fever and what they call in the US, where the blood test is the first rather than the weary last resort of the general practitioner, mononucleosis.

The hypochondriac's temporary nirvana is a clinical diagnosis confirmed by blood test of a non-fatal illness which allows him to moan a bit and smile wanly when asked how he is. From that point of view glandular fever is the perfect illness. I walked home from the surgery a happy man.

Three months later a gland in my neck was still up. I went back to the surgery. 'Well, that's glandular fever for you,' Dr Mulligan said, or words to that effect, this being some time before I'd started taking obsessive notes about the progress of my illness. 'It comes, it hangs around for a long while, it goes.'

A month later I went back again. The diagnosis was the same: glandular fever had become persistent glandular fever. A visit later it was chronic glandular fever, and the visit after that it was about to be whatever the seven month version of the disease is called, when Dr Mulligan remembered something.

'You're on BUPA, aren't you?'

Three years before my father had had the first of a series of heart attacks. The National Health Service did him proud: the ambulance turned up quickly, the emergency team did all the right things, the medical staff looked after him well. At the end of his two weeks in hospital he was told that he needed a routine angiogram to determine the extent of the injury to his heart and that he'd be given it in six months' time. The six months became nine months, a year, eighteen months, two years. It became apparent that the NHS had devised a cheaper and more accurate test than the angiogram: if you lived, your heart hadn't been harmed too much; if you died, it had. Medieval witch-hunters used the same principles when they devised the ducking stool.

On the day when Dad paid for his own angiogram I joined BUPA.

I still like to think that had I not had health insurance the NHS would have given me the same tests I received privately, and with the same promptness, but then again I still like to think that Tottenham will win the double next year.

What a BUPA card shown to a London GP gets you is a referral to Harley Street. Harley Street is where all the private doctors are when they're not being public doctors elsewhere.

London has always had streets which are connected in fact and the public imagination with various occupations. Clerkenwell is for watchmakers, Fleet Street for journalists, Hackney Road for cabinetmakers. Except that none of the connections really works any more. All of the national newspapers moved out of Fleet Street in the early 90s, the quartz movement saw the Clerkenwell watch trade off the decade before and Hackney Road seems nowadays to be a street of pubs and Indian grocers.

C

But Harley Street is still the street of a thousand doctors and has been since the middle of the last century. Almost every one of the tall eighteenth-century houses along Harley and Wimpole Streets and the streets connecting them is the medical equivalent of a brothel: each room is the consulting room of a different specialist and sometimes two or three or more specialists may share the same room, each taking it on different days of the week. On the ground floor is the largest room in the house which serves as the waiting room, its dining table strewn with copies of the various London estate agents' magazines, the sofas strewn with the Arab families and gloomy Russians who seem to make up much of the passing trade.

The rooms look much the same as I imagine they did around 1845 when the doctors started moving in. Some Harley Street doctors are there because they're sufficiently skilful or experienced to have built up a private practice, others because they have the particular diplomatic skills needed to deal with rich, ill people with rich people's special illnesses.

In either case, though, there is some slight and very British embarrassment about the nature of the work they do. God forbid that a Harley Street consulting room should look like a doctor's office; they are laid out as old-fashioned drawing rooms or studies: a leather-topped oak desk, a couple of button-back chairs, some anodyne reproduction oil paintings of the *Fighting Téméraire's* sister ship or the Monarch of the Glen's princeling cousin. And there in the corner, hiding away, will be a tray full of stainless-steel specula or a discreet X-ray light box or a tasteful little ultrasound machine, as often as not stored behind walnut doors in the way they store TV sets in the Home Counties.

A week after Dr Mulligan had passed me over to private medicine I went with my wife to the rooms of Mr Hinton, a dapper Liverpudlian ear, nose and throat man whose business card placed him as a consultant at half a dozen private and public hospitals and who kept rooms at the same address as Dr Mulligan's first choice of specialist.

While Dr Mulligan could refer to the thick wodge of notes which had followed me around the NHS since birth, Hinton knew nothing about me other than what was contained in the brief letter of referral. I told him the story again from scratch – the aches and pains, the glands, the blood test, the lump. And as I told it in full for the first time, I started to worry. As a medical part-work delivered to my own doctor in instalments it had seemed like no more than a catalogue of vague and differentiated symptoms; as a single story it became something else, something with greater narrative possibilities than a mere swollen gland.

I tossed Hinton a couple of possibilities by way of a diagnosis: Hodgkin's Disease, non-Hodgkin's Lymphoma, a few other major, life-threatening diseases taken from the *Hypochondriac's Vade-Mecum* and offered by way of a good luck charm in the knowledge that the true diagnosis is never the one that the hypochondriac suggests to the doctor. It can't be, because the phrase 'That's remarkable! I trained as a doctor for seven years and yet with no training at all you arrived at the correct, and yet unlikely, diagnosis' exists only in the hypochondriac's imagination.

Hinton didn't dismiss anything I'd suggested out of hand. How could he? They'd come from the section of the *Penguin Book of Symptoms* which dealt with lumps in the neck and throat. I had a lump in my neck, *ergo* it could be any of those things.

Hinton felt and prodded and stroked. He sprayed my left nostril with a local antiseptic and passed a fibre optic tube into my nose and down into my throat, following its passage on a tiny TV monitor.

(You want to know the difference between a Harley Street surgery and any other surgery in the developed world? Much later, when I started writing about this, I bought a copy of a 2,000-page American work called *Mosby's Medical, Nursing and Allied Health Dictionary* and a picture book of the thousands of tiny invasive events which can wreck a body. One of the first things I looked up was 'endoscopy' – the procedure which Hinton had undertaken and which would be undertaken again by two more doctors. It shows a photograph of an American doctor looking down a tube connected to a patient's nostril. The American is robed in the full kit: theatre gown, cap and mask. In his discreet Harley Street rooms, Hinton did the job accoutred in a dark blue pinstriped suit.)

We talked for a while about the possibilities and he said that the lump didn't feel like anything nasty, but you could never tell. His guess was a branchial cyst – a cyst caused by a blockage in the vestigial remnant of the gills we had when we still slithered in the Thames mud. It's not a common lump as lumps go, he said, but then again it wasn't going to make the stop press column of the *Lancet*.

He wrote me out three chitties: one to the London Imaging Centre, one to a blood testing lab and one to St George's Hospital.

At the Imaging Centre they'd give a CT scan; at the lab they'd give me a blood test and at the hospital a cytologist he worked with would prick the lump to see what came out. The blood test and the aspiration I could deal with: as far as I knew, though, the scan could only mean he thought cancer was an option.

It was the first time the word had been mentioned in

connection with my neck by somebody who knew what he was talking about.

Even then I wasn't worried too much. I was, after all, in the hands of men with medical degrees and white lab coats. Looking back on my hypochondriasis I realise that I've never been one of those fantasists who wants to be opened up and inspected on a regular basis or even the sort who lives with particular imagined diseases. My hypochondria never demanded more of the medical establishment than that they acknowledge the possibilities of illness from time to time and laugh fondly at my hypochondriacal imagination.

Even on those occasions when my wolf-crying has landed me in hospital – a panic attack in a Soho restaurant, a heart attack while I was filming a TV show on a Yorkshire mountain and which turned out to be constipation – I've found myself laughing alongside the put-upon doctors as if the hypochondria was itself an isolated ailment which we could both inspect together.

I imagined this would be the same.

It was the same, as it turned out. The blood test, at a pay-as-you-bleed medical knocking shop staffed by cool, leggy nurse-receptionists in Calvin Klein lab coats and where the number of credit card stickers exceeded the number of notices referring to medical practice by about three to one, took a matter of minutes.

At the London Imaging Centre the receptionists were less leggy and their white coats were covered in green cardies, but the credit card stickers were still there. They asked for £700 up front and seemed fazed when I said that BUPA would be paying for this. Couldn't I pay them the money and collect it from BUPA later?

C

I don't know why this so offended me: I know, after all, that charging for medical procedures is how the London Imaging Centre pays the bills. I suppose I'd expected something a little more diplomatic – a white-coated flunky who would murmur quietly 'And how will sir be... ahem...' or an invoice posted a couple of days later in a crisp white envelope.

Eventually we agreed that it was unlikely that BUPA would go bust before the bill went in, and I signed something to the effect that if BUPA wouldn't pay then I would.

I was given a hospital gown and a cubicle to change into it, and taken into a room full of a single large white machine with a hole in it.

I'd run my hands over a CT – computed tomography – scan machine before, in the days when they were still CAT – computerised axial tomography – scan machines. The machine is, essentially, a spinning X-ray machine which allows a computer to work out what a cross-section of any part of the body might look like and whether that cross-section might contain anything extraneous by way of lumps, bumps or – who are we kidding here? – tumours.

It was one of the machines that appeared from time to time on *Tomorrow's World*, the BBC wonders-of-science programme which I'd once presented for a while. The great thing about the CT scan is that it looks just like prime-time viewers think the medicine of the future ought to look: white, clean, non-invasive. Press a button and five minutes later you have an instant picture of just what's wrong with the patient. Just like in *Star Trek*.

For five minutes read half an hour, lying stock-still with your head stuck in the machine's cavity; for non-invasive read a syringe full of gunk which heats up the bloodstream and leaves a nasty taste in the mouth. And for instant read when they've got somebody round to interpret the results.

And for reassuring – which all of this was meant to be – imagine the hypochondriac claustrophobe lying with his head enclosed in white enamelled metal, seriously considering cancer for the first time.

Except that I didn't seriously consider it because cancer still didn't come within the remit of my hypochondria in any proper way. Any consideration I could give it was at a sort of existential arm's length. I imagined myself in a week or two's time not as someone who had been diagnosed as having cancer but as someone who had had a close brush with cancer – who'd been through all the tests and then at the very last minute been given the all clear. If anything it sounded even more heroic than the real thing, a sort of *Death of Chatterton* except that Chatterton gets up off the *chaise-longue* to write about it after the painting's been varnished.

Perhaps I was the wrong sort of hypochondriac – the sort who only over-worried about illnesses which could, by some stretch of the imagination, be reasonably feared. Certainly, I now realised, I wasn't the sort who searched through medical books looking for illnesses of which to accuse my body. And as I came to think of it, I realised that still my only real fear was the heart attack, which given my smoking and stress records, was reasonable. Then again, given those records, so was cancer, and still it didn't frighten me.

A couple of days later the blood and scan results came through. Both were negative. There was one test left: the swelling was to be aspirated, which is to say that a cytologist – a cell specialist – would stick a needle into my lumpy neck and divine from the result what the contents might be. Hinton wanted a colleague at St George's Hospital in Tooting, South London to do the job and

C

so I had to wait a week or so until she came back from holiday.

And still I wasn't worried in any real sense. Not as worried, at least, as my wife. Nigella's mother had died of cancer when she was 48 and Nigella 25; 30 months before our trip to Harley Street her beloved younger sister Thomasina had died of a breast cancer which had been shoved into what seemed to be safe remission a year or so before it flourished again. Nigella herself had annual check-ups at the Royal Marsden Cancer Hospital in Chelsea: she was accustomed – if that's the word – to the diagnosis.

It meant that when we turned up at the bright cytology lab at St George's Hospital I was in a calm, 50:50 sort of state while Nigella was holding the arm of a potential cancer patient. Another potential cancer patient.

Here, at least, we'd know immediately what the answer was. Hinton had told us that – more or less, give or take – if the centre of the lump was fluid-filled it was almost certainly not cancerous. What we had to hope for was that Hinton's friend got her lab coat wet. Which she did. The needle went in, a stream of yellow matter squirted out. I was cancer free: a man with a branchial cyst which, when I could get round to it, I should have removed.

The problem was that having it removed would have meant a general anaesthetic and I have an irrational fear of general anaesthetics. And not so very irrational, come to that: people, middle-aged male people especially, go under the anaesthetic and don't come round again. I forgot about the lump.

Or rather I forgot about it as much as I could. I did a TV series in the summer and autumn of 1996 which involved rather a lot of camouflage work on my neck by the make-up artists at Granada. And then one week in February 1997 I sat down in a

BBC radio studio and apologised to the engineer who was about to set up my mike: I was, I said, a bit on the raspy side. It was OK, he said; they were used to it. And I realised that I'd been making the same apology for croakiness for the whole of a 12-week series.

In March I went to New York for a few days. The trip was nominally a work event – I was meant to be writing a piece on the New York press but it didn't much matter whether it got written or not, and the truth was that the reason I'd gone was because I'll always take the opportunity to spend a couple of days in New York by way of a rushed health cure.

This time the cure didn't work. I spent my time there feeling miserable and lethargic. An Internet correspondent who knew about these things had warned me that while a branchial cyst wasn't of itself dangerous, it could become, as he'd put it, 'a focus of infection' and this was precisely what it seemed to be doing. I was coughing, hoarse, unable to eat anything chocolaty or sugary because those substances seemed to burn the back of my throat. I determined that as soon as I got back to London I'd book in for the cyst to be removed.

I got home on the Wednesday and, used to the NHS's way of doing things, assumed I'd have couple of weeks at least before the operation. This was BUPA, though, land of I-need-it-now, and I had an appointment with Mr Mady the next day and was booked in for surgery on the following Monday.

I'm still not quite sure why I finished up with Mr Mady. As far as I could gather at the time, in the months that I'd been putting off the anaesthetic, career paths in South London had changed in some subtle way and I had become somebody else's fee. Given that I had no way of knowing whether Mady or Hinton were any good, and given that the amount of surgery we were talking

C

about here didn't seem to demand a Christiaan Barnard, it was all pretty academic.

Mr Mady had his rooms not far from Mr Hinton's. He was a pleasant enough bloke, as keen to talk about his daughter's gymkhana prospects as he was about my lump. He prodded it, looked down my throat, agreed that it was a branchial cyst and that whipping it out was a matter of an hour's work. Why did I want to go to St George's Hospital? he asked. The truth was because I didn't really trust private hospitals if anything went wrong. Private hospitals are wonderful places if you're slightly ill and need a reasonable hotel with nurses in attendance, but they tend to come second best *in extremis*. The problem with NHS hospitals was always that they started with emergency procedures as the core service and then built outwards. It was bad news if you needed a hip replaced or a varicose vein drawn out, but made sense when your heart suddenly failed under a general anaesthetic.

And so, next Monday I found myself with Nigella in Tooting again, where it turned out there wasn't a bed for me in ENT after all, and did I mind a bed in a ward on the other side of the hospital?

I sat in the day room with my lap-top on an old table and I wrote my *Times* column. It had to be written and I didn't imagine I'd much feel like writing it over the next couple of days; in any case this was as reasonable a subject for the column as any. The column appears in the paper's Saturday magazine, its jaunty title, 'Something for the Weekend', being a remnant of its origins as a column in the main paper which was meant to have been entitled 'Sex Life' until my wife took Simon Jenkins, the then editor, out to lunch and explained that she wasn't prepared to have her husband writing a column called 'Sex Life' in the country's paper of record.

'Sex Life' appeared as 'Private Life' and addressed such libidinous questions as whether the receptionists in salesmen's hotels knew whether the pay-per-view video you'd chosen was one of the clean ones or *Hollywood Vixens*. You know the sort of column. By the time it moved to the magazine it had become a general domestic column – a weekly meditation on life as man, consumer, father, husband. You know that sort of column, too.

This is what I wrote in the hospital:

I'm sitting in a day room in St George's Hospital in Tooting.

I'd intended starting this on a more impressive note of pathos: 'I'm lying in a bed in St George's Hospital waiting for the pill which will allow me to deal less anxiously with the fact that tomorrow a man will come and knock me out and carve slices out of my neck which he'll inspect for malignancy' but some conceited traffic accident victim or selfishly relapsing cancer patient sneaked in and took the bed, *my* bed, and so for some hours I've been shuffled from one day room to another, and now it's no longer even day.

At least it's given me a chance to study the hospital's collection of discreet *mementoes mori*. It's not just the leaflets from the local council posted around the place telling you, so tastefully, how to register a death, or the instructions on how to get hold of an emergency priest or a rabbi when the moment comes. It's everywhere. The reception area is piled with old glossy magazines, each one especially selected to remind you of what the worst-case scenario is about hospitals – and, while you're here, the only-case scenario about life generally. 'When You've Got To Go...' a piece on weekend breaks in *Country Life* is headlined, and 'Dead Reckoning' an article on graveyard photography in *Amateur Photographer*. The headlines leap out of pieces on the mundanities of travel and cooking and wine: A GRAVE SITUATION, NO HOPE OF RETURN, HEAVEN CAN'T WAIT.

News update: they've just told me that there is a bed after all. True, it's so far from the hospital's Ear Nose and Throat sector that they might have to reschedule the operation, but it's a bed. On a public ward. And I feel so crass doing the 'What the hell do I pay BUPA all that money for if I can't have a room to myself' shtick in front of a row of patients who have probably been hanging around for months on waiting lists hoping to get a bed in the NHS lottery. But anger overcame crassness and so I've just had one of those Californian arguments with the woman in charge of beds, the sort where I say I realise that it's not your fault, but you must understand that I'm very angry and there's nobody else around to shout at, and where she says that she appreciates my anger, and she is hearing my shouting, but there's nothing really that she can do.

And just before she goes, she smiles in that nursish way and says she's sure everything will be all right. It's easy for her to say: she'll be sleeping in her own bed tonight.

That's what everyone says. I phone up friends and say 'look, you remember that lump on my neck? Well they're cutting it out and the doctor says he wants to take a look around, just to see what's in there, rather like a police diver uses the phrase just before he goes over the edge of the dinghy into the murky and body-ridden lake. And my friends say 'Hey, don't worry. It'll be fine. I know it'll be fine' which is what we all say when we're not quite sure what the right thing to say is.

It would be reassuring if my friends were surgeons, or nurses, or even pharmacists, but they're journalists and radio producers and magazine editors, and what they don't know about surgery would fill two or three large medical libraries. *How* do they know it will be fine, that the lump is just one of those lumps you get from time to time? Not even the surgeon knows that.

I can't even put it down to my normal hypochondria. Hypochondria normally comes in two varieties. The chronic version which turns every twinge into a cardiac event, every spot into a melanoma, every cold into pneumonia, is the worst because of the not knowing. By comparison, the acute version, in which a doctor with a real medical degree tells you that you do have some actual minor illness and that you can look ill when you tell people about it in the pub, is, in its way, rather cheering. But this is beyond those conditions. Nobody can tell me that the fear of being put under for an hour or so while they cut your neck open is an irrational one.

The pill is taking hold. I shall go to bed now. A public bed in a public ward, but one with clean sheets and surrounded by nurses who accept that men who are about to go under the knife get angry. And frightened. Because while BUPA covers most contingencies, it doesn't cover fear.

In truth it was a manipulative sort of column. Everyone I'd spoken to who wore a white coat said this wasn't about cancer at all. Every test had come back negative. Any fear I had of the lump turning out to be malignant was an entirely manufactured one: hinting that I was afraid of cancer made for a better column than saying I didn't fancy a sore neck for a few days.

At this point I'd had cancer for something over a year.

They cut me the next morning, they stitched me up, they came round that afternoon to tell me how well things had gone. The cyst, the registrar said in that way they have of suggesting

C

you've conspired together to do something clever, was the size of a clementine. It was a woody old thing, full of liquid, and looked benign to the point of saintliness. I slept, I woke, Nigella took me home.

Two days later I picked up a message on my answer machine. Would I phone Mr Mady as soon as possible. My first thought – but not my second – was that this was some sort of procedural problem, that BUPA weren't paying up or that I hadn't signed something at St George's. I phoned Mr Mady's secretary at St George's who wasn't sure where he was that day. I left it. Nigella didn't. Her first thought was different from mine. She phoned every hospital for which Mady worked and left a series of numbers at which she could be reached.

That night I was watching *EastEnders* and waiting for Nigella to come and join me. Ten minutes in she sat down next to me, put a cup of tea down, took my hands in hers and said:

'Mr Mady phoned. He says they've found some cancer cells.'

Well, of course they had.

Chapter 2

C

In its own microscopic way, becoming cancerous is about the most glamorous and successful thing a cell can do.

When sperm meets ovum and life starts, the new cells are the great generalists. As the cells start to divide and re-divide each cell is the same. And then as our bodies, our skeletons, our organs take on shape, the cells start specialising and become, as they say in the trade, differentiated. They know what they are meant to be because only the relevant genetic information is revealed to them. Like the aristocracy; they have no choice, only hereditary duties.

With a couple of exceptions an ordinary, non-cancerous cell is a plodding drone of a thing: specialised in its job of being a liver cell or a brain cell or a skin cell, it beavers away for its genetically allotted span, reproduces itself by splitting into mother and daughter cells, dies. And the cells know when to die because in every one of them are structures called telomeres. A telomere works like one of those old-fashioned calendars they once used in movies to indicate the passage of time. You pulled the pages off one by one and when you got to the last page, that was it: end of the year. Similarly with telomeres: at each cell division, a piece is pulled off the telomere until finally the telomere is just a stub and the cell will divide no further.

This tedious life and death destiny isn't enough for the cancerous cell. The cancerous cell wants to go places, do things that its parents never had the chance to do. A cancer cell is the one that never grows up. The metaphor isn't a casual one: the cancer cell bears all the nastier traits of reckless youth. It defies order, goes where it likes and above all believes itself to be immortal. Indeed, in practical terms the cancer cell would live for ever were it not that doing so does away with the host upon which it needs to live. Cancer cells somehow lose track of what

C

they are meant to be, so when they divide, instead of taking on a sensible function, they become wildly healthy but completely useless and undifferentiated tissue. Which wouldn't be so bad, except they don't know when to stop dividing. The telomeres don't get shorter with each division. The calendar remains forever at New Year's Day.

It's as if these cells, previously healthy productive conformist members of the corporeal society, suddenly – and let us change metaphors here – become members of some wacko religious cult. They become obsessed with immortality and at the same time cease to be of use.

And so the first cancer cell divides and divides and eventually becomes a tumour: a rapidly growing clump of cells doing the wrong job in the wrong place. Again, no problem were the cells happy to stay where they are until the lump becomes visible to the surgical eye – as do the cells in a benign tumour. It can take a cancer cell three years, doubling and doubling in size, to grow to a size where it's noticeable. At this stage the single cell will have become a billion cells. It doesn't take much longer before the cancer becomes fatal – which means that in most cases cancer remains undetectable for 75 per cent of its lifespan.

By the time it's detected, though, it may well be the case that the cancer has started spreading the good word around the body, first locally to nearby lymph glands, and then wandering off around the lymphatic system or along the arterial byways to share the secret of eternal cellular life with other cells in other parts of the body. It invades organs, setting up home there, growing, lumping together, compromising the organ (although rarely actually destroying it) and diverting the body's energies to its own cause.

Up to a point, at least.

Over the next months I would pick up and try to avoid using
any number of jaunty epithets from the cancer set, prime
amongst which would be 'Cancer is a word, not a sentence.' The
corollary of this is that cancer isn't a particularly specific
diagnosis. 'It is,' one doctor wrote to me later, 'rather as if every
viral disease from smallpox and AIDS down to German measles
was given the same diagnostic title.'

My cancer was, said Mr Mady on the phone that night, a
squamous cell carcinoma, an indolent cancer, a cancer which – as
if this would sugar the pill – surprised him as much as it did me.

Not knowing about the 57 varieties, all I heard was that I had
cancer. Mady didn't mention the natural corollary – that I was
going to die soon – but I supplied that for myself. For the one
thing that everyone knows about cancer is that it kills. There is
no curing the cancer patient: the most that can be hoped for is a
temporary remission while the appeal court argues about the
precise date of execution.

Had you told me a couple of months earlier that one evening just
as I was watching *EastEnders* I would get the news that I had
terminal cancer I would have been able to predict my reaction
quite precisely. I would have told you that I would move to the
corner of the room, sit down on the floor and start screaming
hysterically. Something like that, anyway. I've always assumed
that one gets accustomed to one's own mortality at the sort of
age where death as a probability approaches, but I've never been
able to imagine what that accustomed state must feel like.

In the event the terror lasted five minutes, and I have to admit
that even after the first couple of minutes I realised that most of
it was manufactured. I searched within myself for the authentic
voice of dread which I knew must be there, but it wasn't. I wasn't

C

terrified at all: faced with death I was, rather, sad, angry, irritated, apologetic. Sad because it meant that I wouldn't get much more of the plot as it affected three-year-old Cosima and 10-month-old Bruno, angry that it should happen like this and too young, irritated with the frustration of not knowing how to respond, and apologetic towards Nigella who'd had to face enough young cancer announcements already.

Once it became apparent that I wasn't going to scream, I didn't know what to say. What do you say? 'Oh dear'? 'Ooops'? What? I moaned a couple of times, hoping that the moan would encourage the terror to come out of its hiding. I looked at Nigella, and at *EastEnders*, still taking in bits of the plot. I said 'I've got cancer' out loud as if this might explain everything, something. I apologised to Nigella. And that was about as much as I could do. It wasn't as if there were any symptoms to deal with, any evidence of an illness apart from the bandages on my neck. I didn't feel as if I were dying or even as if I were particularly ill.

I could pretend that this serene response represents some heroic act of self-containment on my part, that this was a brave response or a stoical response. It wasn't. It was as involuntary a response as the scream would have been. If it turned out that I was more accepting of death than I'd expected then it was through no fault of mine. Indeed, this may not be the definitive response. It may be that I do recover and that the cancer goes away and that I start screaming neurotically as I once did before I was ill. Or it may be that I buck the odds and die and that when the real final news comes I respond as I expected I would when the first news came. The rule is – and the liberating thing about life-threatening diseases is that they allow one to make up definitive rules about them on the fly – that any response to the news of one's own imminent death is a legitimate one.

At around 8.30 we phoned Mady for an update.

He explained again: this was a squamous cell carcinoma. It was indolent. Translation: squamous cell carcinoma – a cancer of the scaly cells which make up the skin's surface and certain bodily linings such as that of the cervix or the lung or, indeed, the mouth. Indolent: too damned lazy to kill me immediately. There was, Mady said, a high chance of a cure. Surely, I said, he meant it could be put into remission. The other thing we all know about cancer victims is that they are like AA members. Just as an alcoholic is always an alcoholic however long it is since he took his last swig, so a cancer patient always has the killer cells lurking. But no: he meant cured. With the right treatment there was every likelihood that there would be no difference between me and somebody who'd never had cancer.

His opinion was that this was, as it were, a cancer of the cyst. I'd had the correctly diagnosed branchial cyst for so long that it had become cancerous. In fact, he said, the biopsy had found only a few cancerous cells in the cyst and there was no sign of any real tumour. There were a few more in the lymph gland they'd taken out with the cyst, but that was only because the two structures were touching.

He had spoken already to a colleague of his, a Dr Henk, who wanted to see us as soon as possible.

It was late. There was nothing to say. I was still worried that I was feeling the wrong things, that I wasn't depressed or terrified or any of the things I imagined a death sentence would make me feel. The kids were in bed and Nigella and I had no real way to fill the limbo-ish time between now and the next day when I would discover – I hoped – what my legitimate reaction should be to all this.

C

I logged on to the Internet and in a desultory sort of way tried to find out something about what was happening. It turns out that the real function of the Internet, the one which doesn't involve downloading pictures of Korean hookers, is as a resource for the cancerous. The place is littered with sites for the diseased, for their doctors, for their carers. There are sites for people who think prayer cures cancer and sites for those who think acupuncture will do it. There are jolly sites written in the purposeful layman's language of the charitable trust, and furrowed-brow, let's-face-it sites where people get together to wish each other luck. Underpinning them all is the real information – the hundreds of thousands of scientific papers produced around the world over the decades and which sit on the Net waiting to be researched.

I was playing with a whole new vocabulary, though – 'squamous', 'carcinoma', 'prickle-cell' – and one with which I wasn't at ease. In part because both my father and younger brother had been scientists I had a very slightly better than lay command of science writing and indeed, over the years I'd done a little semi-medical writing – consumer pieces on the pharmaceutical industry, columns on the politics of vivisection, sneering pieces about alternative medicine, that sort of thing – but I couldn't make the facts I was dragging off the Net work for me. I had no way to gauge the relative importance of the words I was reading. Was a paper on neck cancers published in Antwerp in 1992 more or less relevant than one on throat cancers published in Chicago in 1987? Was a trial involving 3,000 patients on chemotherapy as important as one involving 200 patients on radiotherapy?

I wasn't ready for this yet. I wandered back downstairs and found a bottle of Bombay gin. It was the first time I'd poured a drink at home for just the two of us in an age but that night we got drunk and hunted out a video which would distract us both.

You would not believe the number of references to death, dying, hell, cancer, serious illness and eternity in *Groundhog Day*. Minute by minute, scene by scene, Bill Murray and Andie MacDowell pranced in front of the snowy Punxsutawney skyline rubbing my predicament in my face in the same way the magazines at the hospital had done a few days before. To the dying all thing are morbid, and I was still dying.

I drank, I took a sleeping pill, I slept.

There was some good news, though. Mr Mady had fixed us an appointment with his oncological partner, Dr Henk. More, he'd fixed it for the next day, which was Good Friday. The bad news, as I read it, was that if an oncologist was willing to come in on Good Friday things must be rather more urgent than I'd been led to believe.

According to Mr Mady, Dr Henk and he worked together all the time. Michael Henk was a radiologist who specialised in irradiating the head and neck and whose main practice was at the Royal Marsden Hospital, a cancer hospital with branches in Fulham and Surrey and a world-wide reputation for clinical and surgical practice and research. Dr Henk is, according to everyone who knows about these things, the best. What he doesn't know about irradiating cancers of the neck is hardly worth knowing: he is one of those doctors of whom one says 'They've sent me to Henk at the Marsden' and watches other doctors nod approvingly.

Next morning we went back to St George's, both of us conscious that with a third visit we were getting too familiar with the place, and met Henk in a small office on the ENT ward.

C

Henk is a middle-aged man with his face set in the tight-lipped and lop-sided smile of one who spends his life leavening good news with bad. We introduced ourselves, shook hands, sat down. Henk looked at his shoes and said 'I'm sorry.'

That's all. 'I'm sorry.' Pause. Tight smile. Look at shoes. Nigella looks at me. I look at Henk. The pause is for ever.

When the man who knows more about neck cancer than anyone in the oncological universe says of the neck cancer which a few hours ago was cheerily pronounced curable 'I'm sorry,' the stomach sinks. I closed my eyes for a moment. Somehow here, surrounded by the piles of sterile wrapped bandages and sutures, the stainless steel hospital impedimenta, the toing and froing nurses, the terminal diagnosis scared me in a way it didn't when I received it at home.

Except that it wasn't a terminal diagnosis. Such is the potency of the word 'cancer' that it can never be delivered without sorrow – even by a doctor who knows the cure rate of this sort of cancer is up there in the 90 per cent area.

Henk explained the cancer in much the same terms as Mady had: a slow-moving, indolent cancer of the neck. Probably.

Probably? Probably is not a word I expect from Mr Neck Cancer. In any case, what sort of probably? Probably cancer? (There is part of me still waiting for the comedy doctor to run on to tell us that there was a mix-up with the biopsies.) Probably slow-moving? Probably of the neck?

The thing is, Henk tells us, that he doesn't really believe in what I'd come to think of as cancer of the cyst. Yes, there are those who believe that a benign cyst can develop cancer but he is not among their credulous number. He conjured an almost medieval picture of disputative oncologists crowded round a preserved cytological relict arguing the toss about the mythical status of the cancer attached to it.

As far as he's concerned the cancer they found in my cyst and the lymph gland they removed with it, is a secondary cancer, the offshoot of a nearby primary. What they will do, he says, is to go back down my throat with an endoscope and a scalpel, have a look around, take a few bits of tissue out to test for cancer, take it from there. The chances are, he says, that radiotherapy will deal with it.

I booked myself in for the next Tuesday, went home and left an e-mail for Bywater.

Michael Bywater is one of only two columnists to whom I've ever sent a fan letter, the other being Alan Coren who will turn up later in this book. I'm not saying that there aren't those to whom I've meant to send fan letters, to whom I've actually written fan letters and not got around to sending them. It's just that Bywater and Coren are the only columnists who have received fan letters, albeit they may not have recognised them as such given the jealousy of their columnar skills which lay barely concealed under my words of fandom.

Bywater is one of those people who is always just about to become incredibly famous. All over London in gatherings of those to whom these things mean anything, people are saying 'Why have they never given Bywater his own chat show/comedy series/incisive post-modernist culture slot on Channel 4?' They will one day, or ought to, but meanwhile Bywater makes a living as a jobbing newspaper columnist majoring in urban existential angst, and with minor credits in art criticism, computer and medical writing. In a life almost exactly as long as mine he has been an opera director, tabloid hack, executive jet pilot and some odd things involving whips and PVC which I've never enquired about too closely. If I didn't like

C

the man so much I'd hate him with a bitter jealousy.

I first met Bywater in 1980 when a dancer who was lodging with my then wife and me kept on telling us that his previous landlord, some sort of journalist called Michael, was more entertaining, forgiving and generally sympathetic than we were. I saw this paragon's name on the guest list of some press junket or another and introduced myself. Our lodger was right: he was entertaining.

Bywater knows about most things, but one of the few things he's actually got a certificate in to demonstrate his knowledge is medicine. He trained in it at Cambridge on the assumption that he would follow his father into the business and although he got diverted from the job by the Footlights mob, he's kept up with most of the reading.

I e-mailed Bywater with the diagnosis and asked for his take on it. Nigella did the sensible and less modern thing: she phoned him and told him to get round here.

Bywater turned up and went into immediate upbeat mode. Yes it was cancer, but only in a superficial sort of way. 'The great thing, of course, is that you can have all the sympathy of a real cancer.' We poured some gin, and then some more. Bywater said he'd go through the Internet with me and show me how to speak the language of cancer. He pressed a button on my computer: a page from the American Cancer Society flashed on to the screen. Bywater studied it.

'Blah de blah de blah – yes look here: 92 per cent. Not a problem.'

We went through some more pages. The way Bywater explained it, the statistics were such that my cancer had actually extended my life. The principle was that yes, 92 per cent of men with my particular cancer lived for ten years after diagnosis: that included all those men with dickey hearts who keeled over when they got the diagnosis, and all those men who fell under buses in those ten years and all those men who were 75 when they contracted the disease. Here I was, young (as Bywater saw it, but then he was born within days of me) fit, middle class.

I relaxed slightly and poured the last of the bottle of gin.

'You know what I really resent?' I said. 'What I really resent is that I bought these wonderful cigars in the duty free shop at JFK, and I'll never be able to smoke another one of them.'

'Rubbish,' said Bywater. 'Look, they're probably going to give you radiotherapy, right? Radiotherapy doesn't piss around: it kills off all the cancer cells, including any you got after the original diagnosis.'

'You sure?'

'Positive.'

Nigella came back ten minutes later. She had left me in the hands of a man I'd promised her knew about cancer. She came back to find us both pissed and giggling with nine inches of cigar sticking out of our mouths.

If the statistics are right – and although my personal 92 per cent turned out not to be, there's no reason why the rest aren't – then Joe Besser is personally responsible for my cancer. The last I heard of Joe he was working in the jewellery business in Hatton Garden, but that was 25 years ago. When I knew Joe properly we were both 13-year-olds at the same Jewish youth club in Hackney.

It was Joe who as we were walking along Clarence Road in Hackney in 1965 said 'I've decided. I'm going to start smoking. It'll help me pull. Do it for a few years, pull women, give it up when I'm 18.' We bought a packet of ten Consulate ('Cool as a

C

Mountain Stream') between us, and we smoked.

This is, I suppose, as good a place as any to explain me and Hackney by way of provenance. I'll make it brief.

I grew up in Hackney in what is usually described as London's East End. I lived there until I was 16 and when I left college I went back there to live and teach. I was still living half a mile from where I'd been born when, at 39, and a year after I split from my first wife, I moved to West London.

In the 50s Hackney was still one of London's Jewish areas: the junior school I went to closed early on winter Fridays because 60 per cent of the pupils would have left early anyway. I wouldn't have left early: although I occasionally took school lunches from the Kosher School Meals Service which existed then and may, for all I know, exist still, I was a secular Jew from a secular Jewish household, which is to say that my parents' politics had effectively superceded the faith of their forebears. Not so very fore, either: while my mother's father, a Stepney barber, had never, so far as I know, practised Judaism, my father's father was a big cheese in the Liberal synagogue.

My parents' vaunted secularism didn't have a lot of effect. True, I wasn't bar-mitzvah'd and am lost at any sort of religious service, but I am in all other essentials Jewish by osmosis if not by practice. In Hackney in the 50s the local vicar was Jewish by osmosis.

We lived on the Webb Estate, a council estate in Lower Clapton. There was a time when I used to describe myself as the product of a Hackney council estate and, leaving the description unqualified, let it offer testimony to my working-class roots. In fact it's been a while since anyone in my family did manual labour. My great-grandfather owned a chain of Yiddish theatres in the East End albeit that he pissed them away with whiskey.

His son, Alf, my grandfather, ran away from home to join the Communist Party and became a book-keeper for the import-export agency which served Soviet Russia as a covert embassy before Britain recognised that state's legitimacy. The agency got raided by the police and Grandpa found himself on what the family always described as 'a black list' although until I wrote the word just now it didn't occur to me how difficult it would be to blacklist book-keepers.

Whatever: eventually Dr Simpson of the eponymous Piccadilly clothing store gave him a job and by the time my grandfather died he was a director of the company. My maternal grandparents were no hornier-handed: Grandpa Hiller was a barber who owned and ran various East End barber shops and who in the 30s started making his own unguents which he sold under the name Rosilla, after his daughter – my aunt – Rose Hiller.

It wasn't as if my parents were *déclassé* throwbacks either. Mum got a scholarship to St Martin's School of Art just after the war and became a clothes designer, and Dad, who dropped out of a degree course at around the same time, was a senior research biochemist who wrote textbooks on the subject and finished up running the biochemistry department at the Royal College of Surgeons.

We were unlikely council estate tenants, but the fact remained that I and both my brothers were born on council estates and lived on them until we were teenagers. It was in part because for all my parents' professional status neither of them earned a lot, and in part because my father's political puritanism didn't quite approve of individual home ownership. Happily he eventually managed to square his conscience and his bank manager and in 1969 we all moved out to suburban Woodford Green where both

C

of them still live.

So: there's me and Joe Besser with our ten Consulate trying to pull. It worked for Joe, but then Joe didn't need the outside agency of cigarettes. I was different. The reason that 30 and some years later I can still remember so precisely the conversation we had that night in Clarence Road is because there is some unreconstructed part of me which still believes what Joe told me then. I don't think that in any literal way smoking helps me pull, but I still believe that I look cooler, more assured, more *me* with a cigarette in my hand – and never mind that I know they stink, I know they kill.

It took me a while to get up to nicotinic speed from the ten a week smoked behind the youth club, but by the time I was earning a living I was on a pack a day. By the time, in my mid-30s, that I took an hour to get my breath back after playing ten minutes of an office football match and decided to quit, I was on two packs a day.

Not that I ever did stop smoking properly. Instead I switched to Nicorette – the nicotine chewing gum. I became addicted to it instead and by the day of diagnosis had been chewing the gum for something over ten years.

I can't tell you that the smoking was definitely responsible for my cancer. I can tell you that 90 per cent of all such cancers occur in smokers. I've had dozens of letters from armchair libertarians telling me that I shouldn't blame the cigarettes because their old auntie died of cancer and she never smoked so much as a Christmas cheroot. Maybe, but they really shouldn't confuse their impotent libertarian argument with the epidemiological one. By all means campaign for some phantom 'right' to smoke, but don't believe that right derives from corrupting the statistics about what smoking does to you. Understand it for what it is: the right to play Russian roulette, as I did, with the immune system.

I woke up the next morning hungover, numb, entirely unready for the biopsy, and with a column to write. The problem was the column I'd written the week before and which was based on the assumption that it was a one-off. I decided that I'd have to confess all:

The me you meet here isn't the real me. He looks much the same as the real me, has the same number of wives and children, combines wit and witlessness in roughly the same proportions, has lived much the same life in many of the same places, but you will understand that if each week I were to deliver to you my life unpasteurised and absolutely as I experience it then that life would be unliveable.

There are, I know, domestic columnists around whose relationship with their partners, their parents, their cleaners and other walk-on characters is so mature – or possibly immature – that they can report every detail of it unfiltered for public inspection and be on speaking terms with their subjects at the end of the exercise. Not me. The me you see here is a sort of parallel me, cravenly picking and choosing the details which will best make the point, changing names or job titles out of a sense of propriety or social cowardice, baring a virtual soul and taking risks only where no risk really exists.

Until last week.

Six months or so ago I wrote about the lump in my neck. I started the piece with a disingenuous reference to an illness which might or might not turn out to be something nasty, and finished it with a smug punchline which, looking back at it now, sneered at anyone who might have been worrying for 800 wordsworth of affected angst whether they were watching a man whose head was about to clunk insensate on to the keyboard.

And then last week I tried the trick again. I'm not quite sure what I wrote because I dispatched the words only a couple of days ago, and because I really did write it in the hospital ward I don't have the piece to hand. But I seem to remember leaving my readers with unanswered questions in the full expectation that at the end of some inconsequential column or another this week I'd note that, by the way, and thanks for asking, but I came round from the operation and everything was fine. I was frightened, sure, but the fear I wrote about was, I now know, the ersatz version which one knows will pass with its cause.

At 8 p.m. on the night I am writing this the consultant phoned up with the bad news and what do you know? I had cancer all along. And have it still. The hubris-hating gods, it seems, read *The Times* too.

So here's my problem. Well, not my real problem, which is that I have cancer and may expire before the date printed on the packet, but my columnar problem.

Cancer is a word of such immense potency that one has to be careful how one uses it in a column. I know the disease is nothing special: people die of it all the time and many more live with, and through, cancer, and I may well be one of the latter. I won't know for certain until they've scanned me next week and carved some random bits out of my throat for inspection, one of the many crass jokes of cancer being that in the early stages the diagnosis is more physically painful than the disease itself.

The question is this: is it appropriate to write about one's own cancer in a jaunty weekend column? Of course there's no guarantee that I'll be able to keep up the jauntiness, especially as the various alternative treatments have the side-effect, says my doctor, of 'making you feel a bit miserable'.

So can I keep the jauntiness up under radiotherapy or, worse, if they tell me I've got only another few dozen columns left in me? Should I keep it up?

I am suddenly very conscious of how I look sitting here. Normally any smugness or bravado or megalomania I exhibit in this space and in my parallel persona doesn't worry me too much: claiming a regular dozen square inches in the country's foremost paper – the paper, after all, the gods read – doesn't make much sense if you're not prepared to be those things.

This is a personal column: I can't just pretend that the event which is currently informing everything I think or do doesn't exist. But if the cancer turns out to be curable don't I risk sounding smugger than ever? And if it doesn't – well, what sort of maudlin is that?

Normally I try to address any qualms I have about what I'm about to write before I sit down to write it. This time, I'm sorry, I can't. There you are: the truth, at last.

Chapter 3

On the way back from the meeting with Dr Henk we stopped off at Sainsbury's to pick up some more gin. One of the things Henk had told us was that spirits were 'probably not a good idea' during radiotherapy, i.e. banned, but that the odd half of lager might be permissible. I've never been a boozer but there was something depressing about being one of those men reduced to sipping a medically approved glass of beer each day, even if it was a glass more than I'd normally drink. I was starting my radiotherapy course the next week and I felt the boozing time slipping away.

I returned to St George's a couple of days later for the biopsy. It was a one-day job: into a day bed in the morning, quick general anaesthetic, up and out in the afternoon. The hospital was getting depressingly familiar: we knew its most mundane workings: the coins the car park ticket machine would accept, the opening times of the hospital shop, the short cut from car park to ward. I knew now not to bother asking for a private room or trying the radio switches above the beds which had been installed before the hospital had run out of the money to buy the radio system to go with them when it sold the building at Hyde Park Corner to a hotel company and moved to run-down Tooting a few years before. We had become part of the hospital's daily operation, as it had of ours.

I'd even lost my fear of the operation or, more specifically, of the anaesthetic which preceded it. My unified theory of hypochondriac hubris had taken over: why would I die under anaesthetic when I had all that cancer to wake to?

The cancer to which I woke wasn't, it turned out, that much different from the one I had when I went under. Dr Mady had removed a dozen tiny slices of throat and tongue including the tonsular stub (and who could have guessed there was a legitimate adjective to be formed from the word 'tonsil') left over from my tonsillectomy 40 years earlier. It hurt like hell and revealed nothing by way of more cancer.

That they'd missed the primary site by millimetres is, this far on, neither here nor there. The primary site was well hidden and wouldn't be discovered for another three months.

Already, though, I was beginning to look and, more importantly, *sound* like a patient of some sort, as I'd demonstrate on the *News Quiz* three days after the biopsy.

For me, Radio 4's 20-something-year-old Saturday lunchtime *News Quiz* and my impending appearance on it was a bigger deal than it should have been but that was because it was so securely tied up with my own professional insecurities.

I'd fluked my way into journalism 18 years before all of this. Apart from a week-long sub-editing course in Scarborough I'd taken 16 years ago, the only professional training I've ever had was as an English teacher in the days when you could still get into teachers' training college with five O levels. I'd taught drama and English in a girls' comprehensive school in East London for four years until I inherited a new uncle, a husband for my recently divorced Aunt Miriam. Seymour Friedlander was a Brooklyn lad who'd come over here some time in the 50s, and his job, as far as I could work out, was to make money in as gentle and discreet a way as possible. 'So whaddya wanna do for a living, then?' he asked me one Sunday when we'd run out of bonding small-talk.

I had my living. I was a teacher.

'No, seriously: what do you want to do?'

Fair point. Well, I said, I'd spent most of my time at college running the student newsletter and magazine: journalism, publishing, something like that, might do the trick.

He told me to phone his friend Sylvester Stein who ran a magazine company in the West End. In fact what Stein ran was a newsletter company – the sort of outfit which runs those ads reading 'Yes! You Really CAN Make Your Fortune In Property! RN of Wythenshawe made £2 million in just one day turning his back garden into a National Car Park... get the insider's facts in the *Property Letter'* and on the back of them sold high-priced subscriptions to cheaply printed words of insider wisdom.

I met Stein, who turned out to be an affable South African who'd left his home country in the 50s just this side of being arrested for membership of the South African Communist Party. Over the years Stein's politics had drifted far enough from its roots to allow him to publish half a dozen essence-of-capitalism newsletters and a glossy jogging magazine – he was the fastest over-60s sprinter in the land – and to run various associated businesses. On the basis of a 20-minute interview during which I showed him some illustrations I'd done for a science book my father was planning to write and let him skim articles which had been wisely rejected by the magazines to which I'd submitted them, Stein appointed me Assistant Managing Director.

I started work two months later. On Friday I'd been Head of Drama at Dalston Mount School for Girls; on Monday I was Assistant Managing Director of Stonehart Publications. On Tuesday, when it became apparent there was absolutely no work for an assistant managing director to do, I became a researcher – *the* researcher – on the *Property Letter*. Three months later when the editor left to go and work for the Socialist Workers Party (the company had a tradition of appointing young lefties to run its capitalist guides on the basis, I always thought, that those of us who distrusted evil landlords would suggest nastier things for

C

them to do than genuine supporters of landlordism who'd have to show them in the best light) I took over. Two months after that Bob Troop, the managing editor of the series of newsletters, had to go away for three weeks: he asked me if I'd look after the property column he wrote each week in the *Sunday Times*.

I wrote three pieces for the paper about interesting things suburban couples were doing with their semis and when Bob returned to take back his column I wrote to half a dozen sections at the paper asking for work. I was, I said, the *Sunday Times'* Deputy Property Editor – I was absolutely nothing of the sort – but what I really fancied writing about, I told them, was motorbikes or dance or education. A couple of months later I was working regularly on the *Sunday Times* magazine. And that, my children, is how you get into journalism.

Even then I held two particular journalistic ambitions: one was to appear on *Call My Bluff*, the wordy panel game on BBC 2, the other to be a panellist on Radio 4's *News Quiz*. And some 18 years later, and within weeks of each other, I'd received invitations to do both. It shouldn't have mattered quite as much as it did: by then I had two BBC radio shows of my very own and a CV which listed a dozen other TV and radio series. But these two were somehow special.

In fact I'd been up to Birmingham to do my two editions of *Call My Bluff* a few weeks before diagnosis; the *News Quiz* was booked in three days after the biopsy. I should have made my excuses – they were reasonable excuses, after all – but couldn't bring myself to do so. I had cancer, for God's sake: they owed me this.

It was a mistake.

The *News Quiz* demands spontaneity, speed, a knowledge of what's been in the news that week. Here I was, retarded by the anaesthetic, my throat so cut about that I sounded like a failed auditionee for the Charles Laughton role in the remake of *The Hunchback of Notre Dame*, my knowledge of what had happened that week anywhere but in the St George's operating theatre nil.

We four panellists hung around in the BBC green room with the producer and the presenter, Simon Hoggart, while we waited to go on stage. I didn't know whether to say anything to them. Although I was eventually to make something of a fetish out of talking about my cancer, the first *Times* piece had yet to appear and I wasn't sure of the propriety of telling four people who were about to go on stage and be funny for their living that the fifth of us had cancer.

Especially given that one of those four was Alan Coren who has done for hypochondria in print what Evel Knievel had done for mopeding. Coren was, as I say, the only man apart from Bywater to whom I'd sent a fan letter and the letter concerned part of the same fantasy as appearing on the *News Quiz*. About five years earlier he'd come up to me at a party at the American Ambassador's house and said 'Aren't you John Diamond?' and I'd written to him the next day to say that when I was 16 my idea of the event after which I'd be able to say 'OK God: you can take me now' was Alan Coren coming up to me at a sprauncey party and saying 'Aren't you John Diamond?' and that it was given to few of us to have our fantasies fulfilled quite so precisely.

Two minutes before we were due to go on I tapped Alan on the shoulder. 'Bad news, I'm afraid,' which suggested, I suppose, that I had some bad news for him. 'It turns out I have cancer.'

Alan is a man who once wrote a piece to mark the day when he decided that such was his risk of a heart attack (in real terms, minimal) that he couldn't take a bath with the door locked any more.

C

He was immediately and extravagantly sympathetic and at the same time immediately and extravagantly startled, for the hypochondriacal world is divided among two distinct species. There are those statistically minded types who rally at the news of another's illness because they think it means there's less chance of their being part of the same statistic, on the same basis as the man who takes the miniature toy bomb with him when he flies on the basis that, hey! What are the chances of there being *two* bombs on a plane? The other half of us treat every mention of a possibly fatal illness as a *memento mori*, a reminder that the gods have got our number and that we should never be under any illusions about for whom the bell tolls.

Alan is one of those, I'd guess, although then was not a good time to pursue the matter.

I went on stage to do the show I'd been waiting all my professional life to do, my own private, triumphal Palladium show. As I struggled to get the failing jokes past my scarred epiglottis I sounded like the bastard child of Jack Ashley and Janet Street-Porter.

Everyone was very sweet in the pub afterwards and said they could never have guessed that I'd had my throat scalpelled a couple of days before, but I knew I had to get my hubris sorted out. Did I accept the next *News Quiz* equivalent on the basis that if I turned it down because they'd always ask me again then the laws of hubris dictated I wouldn't be around when they asked me again, or did I turn it down because I'd be kept alive to suffer the indignity of not being asked again?

Either way round the prognosis remained the same. I had cancer and they had to find a way of getting rid of it.

There are only three interventions which can get rid of existing cancer cells: surgery, radiotherapy and chemotherapy, and I phrase all that with some care – 'interventions', 'existing cancer cells' – for reasons other than those of literary clarity. That is to say that if you are a homoeopath, reflexologist, iridologist or otherwise a scatterer of pixie dust among the deserving middle classes, you have just a couple of chapters or so before you need to start composing your outraged letters to my publisher explaining why orthodox medicine has got it all wrong and why a medical regime which came to its Albanian inventor in a dream in 1937 has to be a better bet.

The principles of all three procedures are pretty easily understood. Surgery, which involves cutting, by scalpel or laser, the cancerous cells out of the body in lumps, wasn't an option for me, because there didn't seem to be anything to cut. Surgeons are pretty accurate with a scalpel but nobody's hands are steady enough to cut out tissue by the individual cell – even assuming those cells are apparent.

When Mady and then Henk had given me the original diagnosis it had sounded to my uneducated ear at best an educated guess and at worst, well, an uneducated guess. By looking at the few cancerous cells they'd so far found, how could they know so much about the extent of the cancer, the distance it had travelled and would travel, the likelihood of it not being a primary and of the primary not being immediately fatal?

In fact the explanation was one of those banal, bubble-popping explanations which Holmes gives Watson all the time.

They had found some cancer cells in the cyst and the attached lymph gland. While some oncologists believe in cancers which originate in cysts, the vast majority believe that you'll never find a cancerous cyst without finding - or missing - a primary close by.

C

But they also knew that mine was a slow-moving cancer. It was almost certain that it had started very near to the secondaries. Even so, mine was an occult primary: they knew it had to be somewhere but there was no way of finding out just where it was.

Chemotherapy was out, too.

Nowadays we use the term almost exclusively to describe cancer treatments, but in fact it means no more than the treatment of disease with a chemical agent. In cancerous terms though, chemotherapy means using one or more of a couple of score of chemicals to attack the cancer more or less specifically. Most often the chemicals tinker with the cancer cells' DNA or RNA and thus reduce the ability of these cells to reproduce. As often as not the chemicals interfere with the legitimate activities of healthy cells too, which is why their side-effects can be so nasty. If surgery and radiotherapy failed then the broad, blunt axe of chemotherapy might turn out to be appropriate, but it would mean that I was no longer a man with a 92 per cent chance of recovery, and at that point, in April 1997, nobody was suggesting that this was anything but a little local cancer which could be polished off in a matter of weeks.

No: I was down for radiotherapy.

Radiotherapy is one of those cures which manages to combine the images of everything which is best and worst about modern medicine. On the one hand it is so obviously modern, involving vast sleek machines which are controlled by computer. On the other hand it equally obviously has its roots in an earlier medical age when the newly harnessed electromagnetic and radioactive forces were applied apparently randomly to recalcitrant illnesses. To hear radiotherapy described in crude terms is like hearing about top-hatted Edwardian physicians giving electric shocks to lepers.

In fact radiotherapy is both crude and refined: crude in terms of what it is, refined in terms of the precision with which it's applied. Simply put, the therapee is strapped down to a bench and has beams of radiation fired at his cancer cells. Or, rather, at where his cancer cells are believed to be. If the radiation could be so finely tuned that it hit only the cancer cells this would be a perfect treatment indeed. As it is, the radiation is fired in the general area of where the radiologists think the cancer probably is. And the cancer isn't just a homogeneous lump but clusters of cells within and around and next to healthy cells.

Thus the healthy cells get zapped too. Indeed one of the principles of radiotherapy is that the go-getting, fast multiplying cancer cells are rather more susceptible to irradiation than are normal non-cancerous cells. A burst of radiation will damage both cells but the healthy cells will recover.

Well, up to a point anyway. For it was with radiotherapy that I would first discover the principle of gradual disclosure which almost all doctors practise.

The principle is simple and at first glance makes a certain sort of sense. In the case of complicated, possibly fatal and emotionally charged illness, never tell the patient more than he is likely to find out for himself, and only ever give the best-case scenario. Thus when we first talked about radiotherapy we were talking about a simple procedure with very few side-effects. When we were discussing occult sites for my primary tumour we were considering a place which almost certainly would not exist after the radiotherapy. When, some months along the line, the subject of surgery came up it was an in-and-out snip-snip sort of surgery.

But the radiotherapy turned out to have a mass of side-effects,

C

it didn't kill the primary and it would lead to eight hours of major surgery.

Meanwhile I had news to break.

I told my parents on the second night. Nigella and I had talked about holding back from telling them for a while on the grounds that we didn't yet know the full ramifications, but there seemed little point in waiting given that even when we knew the full story we knew it wouldn't start with the words 'speaking as somebody without cancer...'

In any case Dad would understand. He might even be able to help. He had, after all, once been a cancer researcher himself once. The first thing I ever knew about cancer was that Dad had once done some research on it for the Imperial Cancer Research Fund and discovered you could get cancer from eating burnt toast or peanut butter. Or possibly it was burnt toast *and* peanut butter: at the time it didn't matter. The burnt toast and peanut butter line was just one of those things we repeated as we took another long toke on a Capstan Full Strength to demonstrate that cancer was an arbitrary sort of hunter down of men and that as there was nothing much you could do to avoid it you might as well smoke 40 a day and take that job in the asbestos factory.

Except that in Dad's day – which wasn't so very long ago – cancer really was a killer. It still is, of course, but in those days a cure was rather more a matter of luck than it is now. Cures involved dreadful toxic chemicals but without the relief of modern anti-emetics and analgesics. There was chemotherapy, but it wasn't focused in a way that some chemotherapeutic regimes now are. And there was radiotherapy but no way of focusing the radiation on precise parts of the body.

What Dad heard, then, was much the same as I'd heard when I

first had the conversation with Mady. His son was going to die.

In fact whatever I was doing by way of repression, Mum and Dad turned out to be able to do tenfold. Or at least that's what they were doing in my direction. For all I knew, at home they were having full and frank discussions about my neck but when they saw me for the first couple of weeks we didn't have a single conversation which didn't have them minimising the threat, the difficulty of the cure, the length of time it would take for me to get better. It was understandable enough, of course. What was happening seemed unlikely enough to me: how much more unlikely would it seem to those two who, inasmuch as they considered the matter at all, had assumed absolutely, and for so long, that they would predecease me.

And in return for their self-protectingly minimising the illness, I would maximise it, scaring them even more than was necessary. Conversations between us became bizarre with them taking about what sounded like a nasty cold and me insisting that death was hours away.

It wasn't until some weeks later when Dad had just told me, again, that some piece of bad medical news was in fact good medical news because it brought a cure closer, that I could bring myself to explain the problem I had with their non-acknowledgement of what was going on. I couldn't really blame them: we are as emotionally as close a family as any I know in all but one respect which is that we don't have the resources to talk about our emotions.

But eventually some two months in I would be able to tell Dad that his denial wasn't helping any. To my surprise he took it on the chin and accepted my point. It was just, he said, that he was scared for me and didn't want to show it. From then on neither of them tried to minimise what was happening, which made

C

it much easier to me to avoid overstating the possibilities.

If at first my parents didn't want to show their fear, there were others who were only too willing.

I've written a column on enough newspapers now to feel genuinely paranoid about the job. Each week for a decade on the *Sunday Times* or the *Daily Mirror* or *The Times* I would send in 800 or 1,000 words of opinion. Of my opinion. In some papers the opinion had been political, in *The Times* it was my opinion about me, about the people I met, the events in which I participated. And I was conscious that interesting as I may have found my thoughts, there was no reason why anyone else should understand why they were taking up space in their paper.

Every broadsheet paper in Britain nowadays has at least one domestic columnist, somebody who sits in the bath and writes a piece which starts 'I was sitting in the bath the other day...' Some of the columns are no more than extracts from a personal diary, others attempt to move from the specific to the general and make a greater point about modern life as it is lived. I've always tried to do the latter but even so I still have the sneaking feeling that mine is the most self-indulgent of professions. Worse, I'd always suspected that my editor, Nick Wapshott and later Gill Morgan, would eventually wake up and come to the same conclusion.

There is only one trick open to the insecure columnist: write a piece which will attract a few letters. It suggests that whatever the editor thinks, at least there are some readers out there who take you seriously enough to write in about you. And the usual editorial line is that letters of complaint are just as worthwhile as letters of praise. The last time I'd tried the trick was when I was perched on a precarious column at the *Daily Mirror* where a fellow columnist, a shrivelled old has-been of a hack, was daily feeding Robert Maxwell invented stories of my failings. I wrote a piece complaining that the BBC were replacing one Radio 2 presenter with another and asking readers to write to me if they disapproved of this. Thousands wrote in: my office desk was piled with the evidence of my high readership. I got sacked two months later, but that's beside the point.

I'd never tried the same trick at *The Times*, in part because as far as I knew there was no rival columnist poisoning the well for me and in part because I enjoyed writing the column enough to want to carry it on on my terms rather than those of a prodded public.

I'd rung Nick Wapshott at the office on the day of my first consultation with Dr Henk and told him what was happening. Would he mind, I asked, if I wrote about the cancer? I'm not sure why I asked him: except for a period when I'd forgotten what it was I was paid to write about and started sending in strange political pieces, I'd not been required to clear my subjects in advance with Nick for some years. Nick was unhappy about the cancer, happy that I should write about it, and thought there was a chance that the writing might help.

In fact the therapeutic benefits of devoting the column to the cancer hadn't occurred to me: I write about what is happening in my life each week and nothing was more happening in my life than this.

For all sorts of technical reasons I submit my copy to *The Times* ten days or so before it appears on the streets. The piece which I'd cleared with Nick – and the one which appears at the end of the second chapter of this book – had been written when I'd just got the news. I'd since written two more. I'd more or less forgotten about that first column.

I was outside the house on the Monday morning after the column appeared doing something internal to the car. It was up

C

on ramps with the bonnet open, I was clad in oil-stained T-shirt and jeans. A motorcycle courier turned up with a thick package for me. I signed for it and took it back to the car where, at its ramped angle, I ripped open the package. It was a collection of hundreds of letters from readers. To have been at the office on Monday morning they must have been posted on the day the column appeared.

I was stunned. If I'd expected any reader response at all it was a couple of anonymous letters telling me that I wasn't the first bastard to get cancer and to stop making a fuss. After all, if my previous columns about my children and my friends and my navel were self-indulgent, then what was one about my illness?

Instead, though, here were letters from fellow sufferers, from the husbands and wives and parents of those with cancer, from those who had once had cancer and been cured, who'd had loved ones who'd died of cancer. There were home-made get well soon cards (who would have guessed that *Times* readers cut out crêpe paper and sticky-backed plastic to make get well soon cards for columnists they'd never met?) and pictures of young children for whom correspondents said they'd forced themselves to get better. Readers wrote about columns I'd written two or three or five years ago which they still remembered and which I thought just disappeared into the local recycling plant each Monday.

I sat in the car and read them, and for the first time since the diagnosis, I wept.

Chapter 4

C

Bravery isn't what it was. I'd always taken the term to describe the actions of those who had put their own safety or comfort at risk in order to do something on behalf of specific others, or for the common good. Recently though, and with the help of the tabloid press, brave has changed to mean something else. It has become a synonym for poignant suffering and usually suffering considerately undertaken in front of the photographer's lens. The five-year-old leukaemia victim is always 'brave little Linda', the mother who goes on bringing up her children after her husband has died is 'Brave widow Mary', although if the husband has died in the pursuit of some noble cause or another – thumping a mugger, climbing a mountain – she might become 'courageous widow Mary' as if the nature of the husband's death quantifies her own bravery.

The bodyguard whose face was smashed up in the Princess of Wales' car crash returned to Britain and the headlines universally referred to him as 'Brave ex-paratrooper Trevor Rees Jones'. At the time nobody on the press had any idea whether he had borne his injuries with fortitude or wept like a baby every day. But he had suffered and thus he was brave, and never mind that the press reports any number of faces smashed in car accidents without ascribing bravery to their owners. What made poor Rees Jones braver than the other victims? That he was guarding a princess who was killed in the crash? That he was riding in a car driven by a drunk? That his story made the front pages rather than the bottom of page 16?

What is it not to be brave, though? Which is the cowardly five-year-old leukaemic? The one who scrawls a crayoned message saying she can't go on like this, and tops herself? Is the widow who decides that talking to the press isn't necessarily the best thing for the kids less brave than the one with a story to tell?

C

About a quarter of my original correspondents took what I presumed at first to be the same sort of line. I was brave, they said. I was brave to suffer my illness so publicly, brave to break the taboo on talking about cancer. Some of them suggested, in that tabloid way, that merely having cancer attested to my bravery.

Others used the traditional bellicose metaphors: cancer was a battle against an evil foe and one which could only be won by the brave. Defeating cancer was an active rather than a passive affair. I had to think myself better, pray myself better. The whole battlefield vocabulary suggested that the cure for cancer had a moral basis – that brave and good people defeat cancer and that cowardly and undeserving people allow it to kill them. But this is the infantile Victorian language of the good dying young and death transformed into a matter of not being lost but having gone before.

I've seen two people die of cancer in my time: my father's sister, Millicent, who died of stomach and breast cancer when she was 49 in 1983, and, a decade later, Nigella's sister, Thomasina, who died of breast cancer when she was 32. Millicent had a young family, everything to live for and bore her cancer stoically and with remarkable humour. Thomasina was the woman for whom the word spirited was coined. If anyone 'deserved' to defeat cancer it was these two.

I am not brave. Indeed, when I say I am the world's least brave person it isn't false modesty speaking: I know me and you almost certainly don't, and I can't think of a single moderately brave thing I've done in my life. If I could have got through those first post-diagnosis months more successfully by sucking my thumb, or crying or lashing out about me I would probably have done so. It just so happened that sucking, crying or lashing weren't my natural reactions to the diagnosis.

But at the Marsden I quickly understood the temptation to describe as brave that which in reality is something else.

The Marsden – The Royal Marsden Hospital Trust – was Dr Henk's base hospital and the hospital to which my cancerous cells were being transferred. William Marsden was a nineteenth-century doctor and surgeon who founded the Royal Free Hospital, the first London hospital which was not merely free but which, more importantly, demanded no letter from a hospital governor for admittance. The Brompton Cancer Hospital, his second project, started as an outpatients' hospital where, almost uniquely in an age when all illness was the sole province of either physician or surgeon, patients could be treated by both.

The technical terms for the various forms of cancer – carcinoma, sarcoma, melanoma – come from the ancient Greeks, who had some limited understanding of pathology of the disease. It wasn't until 1775, however, that the London surgeon Percivall Pott first described an occupational malignancy – the cancer of the scrotum and elsewhere common in the young boys sent up chimneys by sweeps. It was, although he didn't describe it as such, the same squamous cell carcinoma that I had, and was almost invariably fatal – the qualifier 'almost' covering the few boys who had their cancer cut out, without anaesthetic, who lived through the operation and the inevitable subsequent infection and in whom the cancer didn't recur.

Marsden had better luck. Using new surgical methods he started cutting out cancers and on occasion curing patients. The hospital took his name and, a century or so later, was subsumed into the National Health Service as an oncological centre of excellence. Indeed one can tell just how good a hospital it is:

C

Virginia Bottomley as Minister of Health tried to close it down, and she seemed interested only in closing down the very best medical institutions.

Like many of the best hospitals in British cities, it is a mixture of the ancient and the modern. The hospital sits on the Fulham Road, a couple of hundred yards in one direction from the shops of the King's Road in Chelsea, and in the other from the concentration of Terence Conranism at South Kensington. If cancer were chic then this would be the chic-est hospital in town. The main block is a rather gloomy Victorian mansion, all sweeping staircases and lugubrious portraits of dead benefactors and ramps nailed over the level changes unsuitable for wheelchairs and trolleys. On to this has been tacked a series of more modern buildings in bright brick and straight out of the pattern book of cheery hospitals. Happily for the patients most of the wards seem to be in the new parts of the hospital: it's only in areas like the histopathology department that staff work with the paint falling off the walls.

I'd expected the Marsden to be a depressing place. After all, everyone there has a potentially fatal disease, and while the waiting rooms at St George's were full of men with broken toes contemplating a football season on the injury list, the waiting rooms at the Marsden were full of people contemplating something rather longer term. Or, I suppose, and depending how you look at these things, shorter term

As I queued in the outpatients department for my first appointment with Henk I saw that the woman in front of me had three appointment cards taped together like a jet-setting business traveller with her bundle of visa'd passports. As I waited I worked out from the number of appointment spaces on my own card that she must have been here getting on for 100 times. She was approaching middle age, well turned out, hair bobbed, clothes Marks and Spencer trendy. But after 100 visits to deal with her recalcitrant condition she looked no less apparently cheerful than any other queuing Briton. No less cheerful, indeed, than the dozens of outpatients waiting their turn in the reception area, every one of whom had cancer or was a relative or friend of someone with cancer. The waiting room should have had the atmosphere of a modern death row without the blues harps and the tin cups, and there's no doubt that for all that these people have learned the cancer ward's new rubric – 'Cancer is a word, not a sentence' – some of them would die of their illness, and soon. You'd never know it, though, even if the place does have more than a normal hospital's share of outpatients with bits of their face missing, or the obvious reactions to chemo- or radiotherapy.

I've never been one for going gentle into that good night, and I don't know whether the Marsden's cheerfulness says something about the average Briton's craven acceptance of everything that's thrown at him, as if an early and painful death is something which, like bad service at a restaurant, shouldn't be complained about too loudly in case anybody sees you making a fuss. I'd prefer to believe the cheerfulness is down to the hospital itself. The Marsden is the most cheerful hospital I've ever been in, and it's not the relentless spit-in-the-face-of-adversity cheeriness either, but a genuine mixture of realistic hope on one hand and efficient expertise on the other.

A couple of days later, and back for some radiotherapeutic preparation, I found myself next to a woman, capped to hide her baldness, hollow-eyed, dressed in clothes which probably fitted snugly a month or two before and which now gaped and sagged. She'd fallen down some stairs at the office, she said, and went to the doctor when the resultant bump at the base of her spine wouldn't go away. It turned out to be some sort of spinal cancer: she'd had chemo and had lost a couple of internal organs and would be travelling in each day from 30 miles away for treatment.

We swapped details about what we'd heard about radiotherapy and in five minutes I'd forgotten that I was talking to somebody who probably wouldn't live to the end of the year. She smiled, she joked, she told stories of medical indignities and deprivations in the way that others talk about the office photocopier breaking down.

I kept on wanting to say, in that newspaperish way, 'My, but you're being so brave' but I didn't. I'd become wary of the word 'brave'. The new, tabloid, brave is an involuntary state but true brave is what you are when you have options, and at the Marsden there are no options. Everyone here could see someone in a worse state than themselves, and with a worse prognosis. And we all knew that given any sort of option at all we wouldn't be there.

If I'd become ill because I'd chosen to take my daughter's illness to save her from it, that might have been brave. But I had no choice. I had cancer and this was how I was reacting to it.

As for my supposed bravery in writing about my cancer, this was way off the mark. I write for a living: I earn the mortgage money translating what I see and hear and feel into words on the printed page. And while I've never been convinced about the service I thus provide to the public, I know, as does every third-rate psychotherapist, that writing things down helps. Who, given the opportunity and the diagnosis, *wouldn't* want to write about it?

(Lots of people, as it turns out: I've since come across any number of journalists and writers who suffered cancer and worse and were never so tasteless as to bring the matter up in print. Some of these regret that they couldn't do so, others can't understand why I would want to and a third group seem to feel that whatever my motives for wanting to I should suppress them in the name of British good taste.)

As for breaking the taboo, well the simple fact is that I didn't know there was a taboo about mentioning cancer. This probably has something to do with the Jewish thing for I come from a culture where all illnesses – colds, flu, bowel complaints, cancers – are discussed interminably and without any reserve.

But the letters told me otherwise. Now I came to think of it, of course, I realised that cancer was a disease more beset with euphemisms than any other. These days we understand the word 'tumour' to be synonymous with cancer: in fact it simply means a swelling and was introduced into the medical vocabulary by doctors who couldn't bring themselves to use the word 'cancer' in front of the punters. These were the doctors about whom my correspondents wrote. There were letters from people whose parents had died of cancer without the word ever being mentioned to them, people who'd had malignant tumours cut out by surgeons who would only ever talk about 'a bit of a lump', people who were now on heavy-duty chemotherapy but whose relatives would only ever talk about them being 'ill'.

Which is not to say that I wasn't having problems talking about my own cancer.

It is not a matter of taboo but of simple etiquette. You get to a certain age, you assume you've got a handle on most of social intercourse's more likely eventualities. After a few false starts you've learned how to do sending the meal back, dropping the girlfriend, getting through the job interview, making the marriage proposal: you think you've got it taped. And then one day some new circumstance pitches up and you realise that you're not, after all, living the life you thought you were living, and that there are some quite basic exchanges you don't know how to do.

And so in the days between diagnosis and the first column appearing, a friend would phone up and ask, as is the way of these things, how I am. Sometimes I would forget how I was: I'd say, as one does, 'Fine, and you?' and then have to backtrack, because of course I wasn't fine. So I'd say 'Actually, I say that, I say I'm fine, but, well, I've got cancer.'

What else can you say? You can't build up to it slowly – 'I'm ill. No, not a cold: really ill. No: worse than flu. No, no: better than AIDS but worse than flu. OK: two syllables...' – or drop it casually into the conversation – 'Things? Things are so-so, you know? I got the new computer, and somebody smashed the car window and nicked the stereo, and I've got throat cancer, and we thought of going to see the new Tarantino, but...'

And then there's the question of making the announcement appropriate to the person you're talking to. I didn't want to make too big a deal of it – 'Look, perhaps you should sit down for a moment, because there's something I have to say...' but then again I didn't want to minimise the situation – 'Nah! Just a little thing, you know? Six weeks, all over, don't even think about it' – because it didn't feel minimal. And then there were people who weren't close or who were on the periphery of my professional life and who would need to have the information, but from whom I couldn't expect the same sort of reaction as I could from proper friends. I tried telling this group merely that I wasn't too well at the moment but as often as not they'd push: when would I be better? when could I get back to them with the figures? couldn't they just send a bike round for the copy?... and I'd have to tell them what sort of not-too-well I was and they would get terribly upset because on the one hand they were sure they'd said something inappropriate to such an unmentionable illness and on the other hand they felt that I'd somehow suckered them into their inappropriate response by not telling them straight off what the deal was.

So I'd just say I'd got cancer. In any case for the first few days I said it as often as I could, because I still didn't quite believe it. Nigella and I would sit in the consultant's office surrounded by chatty leaflets on nausea in chemotherapy and say to each other 'What are we doing here?' But even if I got used to the idea I never found a truly satisfactory way of announcing it to others.

By the second week I decided that the best way was to come straight out with it.

'John? It's Charlie. How are things?'

Oh you know things. I've got cancer.

'You're joking .'

No: I'm serious. I've got cancer. They told me last week.

'Jesus. I mean... Jesus. So what is it?'

Throat. It was that lump I had.

'Yes, I remember it. So... you know... how... when does... do...'

They reckon they can cure me. It'll mean six weeks' radiotherapy but there's a pretty high cure rate.

At which point the conversation goes one of five ways. The first is when they confuse radiotherapy with chemotherapy and start commiserating with the sickness I'll feel. That's easily dealt with.

The second is when they think that my report of the high cure rate lets them off the sympathetic hook.

'Oh, that's OK then. You gave me a bit of a scare. Whew! Look, about that book you were going to sort out for me...'

C

·I'd always feel short-changed after one of those conversations, as if the cancer was being taken away from me. Yes, it was one of the safer cancers but it wasn't a cold, for Christ's sake. (There was an element of hubris at work here too, of course. If I started telling everyone that I'd certainly be cured then I almost certainly wouldn't be.) I'd explain that this was real cancer, just like the cancer that killed people, and that it might kill me. They would apologise for their oafishness at mentioning the book and start asking sympathetic questions about my real cancer, and then I'd feel guilty at making them feel guilty and would say no, look, about the book... and so we'd go on, round in circles.

The third line was the 'you'll get better – I know you will' one which I'd encountered before the first operation and about which I'd written in that first column. It was bad enough when it was just a matter of recovering from a cyst but when they were giving their judgement on throat cancer I started to get angry.

'John – it will be fine. I know it will.'

How do you know?

'Because I know *you*. You won't let it defeat you.'

You know me? What, you know that I'm immortal? That I'm not susceptible to cancer like other people?

'No, just that, well...'

It was unfair of me, I know. People say things because they don't know what to say, and they turn their wishes – that they don't want me to be ill, to be frightened, to die – into statements of fact. I would tell other friends how irritating I found the you'll-get-better set and they'd say 'Yes, but you ought to indulge their fear', which seemed an odd demand to make of me: I had cancer and yet I had to indulge others in their fear of it.

Eventually, though, and over the months to come, I learned to indulge and they learned that wishing the cancer away wasn't a recognised cure for the disease. Or, at least some of them learned it, because there was a fourth group who were the most irritating of all.

'John, Charlie told me the news. It's terrible.'

Well yes, it's pretty–

'I can't tell you how dreadful I felt when I heard. I had to take a Valium, of course, because you know what I'm like, and that was the afternoon gone. I couldn't write a thing.'

How dreadful for–

'I know. I know. It ruined the day and then I went to Fiona's party in the evening and everyone asked why I was looking so miserable and I told them, and they couldn't believe it, and I'm afraid it threw a bit of a pall over the whole party, because it turns out that Eddie's father had the same sort of thing a few years ago and he got glum telling us about it...'

Of all my friends, the set who wanted a go at vicarious cancer and who insisted on telling me how painful my cancer was for them were the ones who, over the months, I fell out of touch with.

The fifth group, which is to say the rest, were, well, remarkable. I determined pretty early on in all of this that I wouldn't fall sucker to the ill-wind fallacy. I have met people who have told me that they are in some way better people for their brush with cancerous death and that looking back on it they were glad they'd been hit. And I have to admit that when I discovered that my reaction to the original news wasn't the hysterical one I would have imagined for myself I began to see a positive side to the experience. But for all that, and for all the other paradoxical benefits that cancer has brought, I cling to the belief that anything which stops you kissing your children goodnight or telling them a story – and both eventualities would happen soon

C

– has to be, on balance, a bad thing.

But having said that, there is something moving in discovering that you have friends who say 'If there's anything I can do...' and who really mean 'anything'.

Dr Henk talked me through the radiotherapy. He wanted to get it started as soon as possible. He made this urgency sound a matter of convenience – 'The sooner we start, the sooner it's over, you know?' – rather than one of medical expediency. He had seen me for the first time on Good Friday: the therapy was to start on the first day of Passover just three weeks or so later.

Henk still had no precise idea where the primary site of the cancer was, but knew that it was almost certainly close to the cells they'd already removed. I'd had a second series of the tests that Hinton had ordered back in 1996 and no abnormal mass had shown up on either the X-ray or the scan. I'd always understood that the magical CT scan hunted out cancer however small it was: it turned out that nothing smaller than a centimetre or so shows up on a scan, and that even a reasonably sized tumour may not always be apparent.

As he explained them to me the chances were, then, that the primary site was a small one. In fact around a third of primaries in my sort of situation were never detected but were wiped out by radiotherapy. He hoped mine was one of them. As, of course, did I.

He wanted to irradiate the left side of my neck from just below my ear to level with my chin and the left side of my throat. If I'd been in America, he said, he would have treated both sides of my throat as a matter of course but then Americans were neurotic about such things and in his experience there was no point in having radiotherapy's side-effects on both sides of my head unless it was absolutely necessary.

Ah yes: the side-effects.

What could he tell me? There'd be a bit of soreness to the skin – the sort of thing you get if you stay out in the sun for too long, but it would be temporary. And there would be a sore throat, of course, but that would be temporary too. And I'd lose my saliva glands on that side of my face.

'Temporarily?'

'No; for good, I'm afraid.'

Well nothing too bad. But then I'd forgotten about the principle of gradual disclosure. A couple of days later a registrar said in passing that of course I knew, didn't I, that I'd lose a bit of hair round the radiotherapy site.

'How much hair?'

'Oh, you know. Just a bit at the collar-line.'

And as he said collar-line his hand traced a line along the back of my head just about the ears.

'Permanently?'

'No, no. Temporarily. It'll come back in four months. Just like your beard. Probably.'

And then the next day Henk asked me if I'd booked in for my dental treatment yet. My dental treatment?

It turns out that one of the side-effects of radiotherapy is the damage it wreaks on the smaller blood vessels and their ability to carry oxygen around the place. It means, for instance, that a tooth pulled from an irradiated jaw will take a lot longer to heal than normal, and may not heal at all. The vessels don't start collapsing until some weeks after the radiation and so, Henk said, it was usual practice to get rid of any teeth that looked as if they might give problems in the future.

'This isn't temporary, then?'

C

'No. Permanent.'

I was given a date with Sarah Howells, the Marsden's dentist, who pulled out a tooth from my lower left jaw and, bless her, laughed at all my jokes. This is what it had come to: as the hypochondria had slipped away in the face of real illness I had turned into a man who could lose a tooth under a local anaesthetic and joke about it as it was happening.

Howells gave me a tube of fluoride gel. I was about to lose half my saliva glands for good. Saliva has a number of functions, one being to help get food down the gullet and the other to neutralise the acidifying effect of that food just like they say in the chewing gum ads. With half my saliva gone that neutralising effect would be reduced and I'd need to rub the fluoride gel into my gums every night.

'For how long?'

'Oh, you know. For the rest of your life.'

There were three stages to the radiotherapy itself.

The first was to get my mask made up. Radiotherapeutic success is based on giving the area as much radiation as the healthy cells can stand and on making sure that the beams are fired into exactly the same area every time. I would be having the standard treatment: 30 daily doses of radiation over a period of six weeks. There are a few ways of making sure the rays hit the spot every time: some involve marking the skin itself but mine involved having a Perspex mask of my face made. The mask would hold my head down to the bench under the radiation gun which would be lined up with a series of marks made on the mask by the radiotherapists.

In the basement of the Marsden I lay down on a table in the mask room while two radiotherapists covered my face first with dental putty and then with two stone of plaster of Paris leaving holes only for my nostrils. It was almost a relief to discover that the cancer hadn't got rid of all my neuroses: I was still sufficiently claustrophobic to balk at the idea of having my eyes and mouth covered with setting plaster. We argued the toss and I persuaded them that if I wasn't being irradiated in the eyes or mouth there was no need for them to take an impression of them.

The resulting mask was a cumbersome see-through version of the black latex hoods they sell in the more recherché sex shops with that same gaping mouth hole and sightless eyes. All it needed was a couple of hooks to take a chain or two.

Next came simulation.

The body is a three-dimensional object and the radiation not only has to hit certain points on the mask but penetrate to a specific depth. In the run of things it wouldn't much matter if it went a millimetre or so deeper than Henk had specified in his guess of the widest area to which the cancer might have spread: the healthy cells would, after all, recover. The trick was avoiding the spinal column, for if that got irradiated then a few months after the last session I would find that I had lapsed into a state of paralysis. Permanently.

The simulation room was down the corridor from the mask room and consisted of a machine very much like the one which would irradiate me, except that this was set up to record the rays that were emitted. For two sessions of 45 minutes I would lie with the mask over my face, unable to move my head, while the radiographers pressed buttons and took measurements and shouted numbers to each other. It was rather like being measured for a very expensive suit with the advantage that here they didn't make worrying observations about the size of my

C

stomach and backside.

Then again, in a week's time the radiotherapy would start and my stomach and backside would shrink to almost nothing. And still I had no real idea of what my chances were, of whether this was a routine method of bringing minor-league cancer patients like me back on to the path of health and longevity or whether it was a fingers-crossed, you-never-know-your-luck punt at trying to save my life. That week I devoted my column to the unknown, unknowable statistics:

I'd intended setting my swollen jaw and gritting my remaining teeth and laying off the cancer this week and returning to the usual, and in particular to the giggling authoress who announced so proudly on the radio that she couldn't ever make a word processor work as if this confession conferred upon her a finer intellectual sensibility than admitting she couldn't tie her shoelaces or open a can of soup.

Had I stuck to my resolution I would probably have gone on to ask at which point it was that it stopped being the vulnerable peasant classes who cowered before technological advance and became the enlightened chatterers who were forever boasting that they couldn't set the video recorder or wire a plug.

And I would have probably meandered to the end of the thesis with the conclusion that, properly dissected, bourgeois technophobia is as much a part of the class war as anything involving Molotov cocktails and badly printed pamphlets, and that what it represents is a resentment of the democratising influence of technology. After all, if the masses can do clever things with cheap computers then computers must be demonstrated to be on a par with...

Well, you take my point. But the resolve faded and that's as far as I could get. Hypochondria took over.

One of the benefits of a proper illness to neurotics like me is that it shows us the error of our little hypochondriacal ways. Once doctors' eyes would glaze over and they'd start doodling on those little pads that the Prozac people give away as we listed the vague and ambivalent symptoms of our vague and ambivalent illnesses. 'Well,' we would start, 'it's not so much a pain exactly as a sort of...'

Since the diagnosis, though, the doctors rush round the moment their bleeper sounds to canvass us for new symptoms. And when we deliver them, they repay us with details of the real illnesses they may represent. Two months ago if I'd mentioned the dull pain in my arm I'd have got a brief, bored lecture on what happens to arms when they get to my age. Now I get a professional wince, a sucking of teeth and talk of a bone scan.

For the first couple of weeks the big illness with its big symptoms and its radical cure put all the other niggling crypto-symptoms into perspective.

Now, I'm not so sure. The problem with illness is that nothing is certain. I started off with a definite diagnosis – cancer – and nothing more than that. Gradually the diagnosis was refined to curable cancer. And then it was broadened out again: curable cancer, provided it's the cancer we think it is and that the bit we cut out contained its primary source.

And all the time there are the qualifiers: the probablys and the possiblys and the weasel statistics which are wonderfully accurate if you're a whole population and meaningless if you're just a single bloke lying under a lump of fizzing Cobalt 90 while the radiographers run for cover behind their lead screens.

And every extra symptom – real, imagined, pre-dating my cancer or newly arrived – changes the odds, and changes them to

C

a number that is unknowable. It is the state that we live in all the time, however unconsciously. But in these circumstances it's difficult not to try and calculate the incalculable odds, and impossible not to want to. 'You'll have to be a bit of a stoic, I'm afraid,' said the nurse as she totted up the side-effects which would accumulate over the course of the radiotherapy. Well, I'm sorry, but if I was a stoic then I wouldn't bother with the radiotherapy at all.

What I need now is a doctor who will tell me that he's run my body through an electronic mincer and can tell me without any doubt that there are this many cancer cells remaining, that they will be killed off on precisely this day, that there are no rogue cancer sites in my toes or my ears or my kidneys, and that Blue Boy will win the 4.30 at Kempton Park.

What I get instead is the same ambivalence I used to offer the doctors in my days as a healthy hypochondriac. How could they possibly offer me anything else?

Meanwhile, I lie here under a few hundred thousand pounds' worth of impossibly complicated machinery while confident and competent women who aren't ashamed of knowing the reason for the constancy of Planck's constant murmur numbers to each other, and I contemplate the crass smugness of the woman on the radio who thinks the smart thing is to believe that technology is for the proles.

Chapter 5

It was when radiotherapy began at the end of April that I started to get ill.

Of course I was already ill, but it wasn't any sort of illness you could put your finger on. I could see now how doctors, never mind patients, could miss cancer until it was too late, until the primary had spawned local secondaries and then set off on the trek to the distant, fatal sites around the body. Had my secondaries not decided to display themselves as a cyst I'd probably still know nothing about my own cancer. Apart from the healing scar around my neck where they'd taken out the lump, I looked healthy enough and in fact I'd even lost some of the usual zombie pallor that I manage to keep even after two weeks in the Caribbean. Most of the time I felt as healthy as I ever did, which isn't, I grant you, saying a whole lot. Indeed, my only symptom when radiotherapy started was hardly one of cancer. It was simply that still, five minutes after I ate anything I'd cough and a small pellet of food which had been hiding in some new crevice in my throat would jump into my mouth. And combined with this, I was still getting the same strange burning reaction in my mouth whenever I ate sugary and, particularly, chocolatey food.

But these weren't symptoms of cancer. At least the doctors at the Marsden, where they knew more about cancer than anywhere else, didn't have them pegged as symptoms of cancer. (This is, as I'm sure you've gathered by now, what we in the narrative trade call dramatic irony. But even so you'll have to wait a couple of months – say a chapter or two – before a surgeon says 'Funny that – you're the third person I've seen recently with throat cancer who complained of that sensation when they eat chocolate.' Funny indeed.)

As things stood, the prognosis was simple and optimistic.

C

They'd found a secondary and six weeks' worth of radiotherapy should, they guessed, clean up the nearby primary. End of story. When radiotherapy finished I'd start on weekly checks for any recurrence, then move to monthly, six-monthly and eventually annual checks. And after five years I'd become a name in an archive somewhere and we could all forget I'd ever had cancer.

Radiotherapy was simple, too. In the basement of the Marsden were two modern, white rooms the size of small barns. Set in the middle of each room was a vast, white Varian radiotherapy console – a slab of a machine with, at one end of it, a head capable of directing consistently finely tuned beams of radiating ions at any part of a patient lying on the bench beneath it. It looks like a very modern, very streamlined version of the machinery a contemporary Frankenstein might use to direct the lightning bolt at his monster.

Being irradiated is, of course, what we spend a lot of our lives avoiding. The radiation which is emitted by these machines isn't so very different from that emitting from the world of machines which have exclamatory yellow labels reading DANGER! RADIATION! DO NOT COME NEAR! HONEST: YOU'LL DIE! WE'RE NOT JOKING. JUST *GO AWAY*, OK? It is the same sort of radiation which saw off – and is seeing off still – many of the citizens of Hiroshima and Nagasaki, and which kept us all awake for so many nights after the irradiation of Chernobyl.

And what is the one thing we all know about this radiation? Of course: that it gives us cancer. So presumably there is a difference between the radiation that gives us cancer and that which cures us of it, right? No: it's precisely the same stuff. Nor are we talking some homoeopathic interaction between disease and cure: radiation cures in just the same way that it kills, by knocking out cells. It all sounds unlikely and indeed it was when

I mentioned in the *Times* column that I was about to start radiotherapy that I began to get the first few letters from that chapter of the anti-medical lobby which specialises in the simplistic connection between what looks a possibility and what is certain.

The small number of anti-medicalist correspondents split first into two groups and then into three more. The first two appeared, as it were, as the benign and the malignant. Benign letters came from those who wished me well but thought that before I went any further I might want to read the enclosed copy of *God's Black and White Salvation Diet* in which slim, self-published pamphlet the German theosophist Hugo-Mannfried Gottmeyer tells how the prophet Elisha had come to him in a vision in 1956 and revealed to him the secret of cytological integrity which lay in eating two bags of liquorice allsorts a day.

The malignant were the ones who told me that as a journalist with a public platform it was my bounden duty to stop operating as a propagandising dupe for the evil medical establishment, to tell my doctors that I wasn't fooled by their fake radiography statistics when everyone knows that radiation kills, and to put my faith in the Bessarabian radish, the desiccated root of which has been used for centuries by Tartar nomads to cure athlete's foot, tennis elbow and cancer, as detailed in their book *Why Your Doctor Hates You And Wants You To Die*, review copy enclosed.

Each group, the demanders and the gentle nudgers, broke down into a further three groups: the religious; those who were well-versed in the lore and practice of alternative medicine; and those who admitted to knowing nothing about science but who knew that homoeopathy had worked when their husband had cancer in 1987.

C

It was this last group to which I had the most difficulty responding. They were usually the kindest and most flattering of correspondents, and I wished sometimes that I could have written back to them and said that yes, I would try their regimes and report back. The problem was that they tended so often to subvert their own claims. I must have had dozens of letters from readers whose alternative therapies worked in all but one respect: they didn't cure the cancer. People would write to tell me that when their spouse had a cancer similar to mine they swore by a food combining diet which had worked wonders all the way to the day, a year later, when said spouse died.

Alternatively they would write to tell me that they had used alternative medicine in conjunction with radiotherapy or chemotherapy and here they were, ten years later, able to tell the tale. Invariably my correspondent would put the cure down to the arbitrarily chosen and applied alternative regime rather than the carefully controlled orthodox regime, but I could never bring myself to write back and ask why, precisely, they thought it was the odd diet which had saved them rather than the radiotherapy.

The most difficult of all to deal with were the religious letters. The first came in the first bundle I received after I outed myself as a Person Of Cancer. 'We are praying for you,' it said, and nothing else. No return address, no signature, no indication of whether I was being prayed for by the quietly murmuring congregation at Westminster Abbey or the Hallelujah-be-praised! set at the Save-A-Soul Mission 'n' Takeaway Grill, Letchworth.

In the next post were a few more letters: one from a family who'd lit a candle for me at Liverpool Cathedral, another from a woman who enclosed a copy of the prayer she had said for me the night before, a third sending a pro forma to tell me that I'd been mentioned in heavenly dispatches from Walsingham. And with every postbag came more prayerful letters. They weren't, for the most part, from religious nutters, but from people for whom religion was as much part of their life as food or TV. Some didn't even go that far but just wrote to remind me that given that nobody knew what was out there, what could the harm be in sending up the odd prayer?

I've always suspected that if there is anything to prayer then it's not something you can start up when times get bad. I don't know how the scheme would work, but what if it's only available to those who kept up their spiritual subscription through the good times? Who knows what the hubristic risks are of drawing on an empty account? Always assuming that a modern Judaeo-Christian upper-case G God has adopted the hubristic notions of the ancient lower-case g Greek gods.

A very few urged me to take to praying myself and one told me sternly that I had no chance of recovery unless I called Doctor Jesus to my bedside. Most, though, showed a greater generosity of spirit: they understood that I might not be a believer myself (some even recalled my occasional references to my own secular Judaism in the column) but that didn't matter because a prayer's recipient need be no more conscious of the deed than is a beer mug of accepting a pint of best.

Some people would send aids to help me pray. I have a rosary made of white plastic, a cross made of olive-wood taken from the Mount of Olives in Israel. Somebody, of less formal religious bent, sent me some wax with instructions on how to make a juju image of my cancer and squish it away.

I even received a letter from that sweetest of men, the Chief Rabbi, to tell me that prayers were being said in the highest quarters. Well, the second highest anyway. My grandfather

C

would have *kvelled*, *kvelling* being the Yiddish word which most precisely describes the emotion of a grandfather on discovering that his cancerous grandson is being prayed for by the Chief Rabbi. There is almost certainly another Yiddish word which describes the act of hypothesising on the possible emotions of dead grandfathers, but it's not one I've yet come across.

This being prayed for was an odd feeling and each time I got a prayerful letter I'd run through the same set of internal responses. First was my customary wonder at the kindness of strangers, second was gratitude. And then came guilt: should an agnostic be accepting prayers? Should a Jewish agnostic be accepting prayers from Christians? Should a Jewish agnostic be accepting prayers from Jews, come to that?

And then came confusion. We are all, inevitably, subverted by our own prejudices, and like every agnostic my fear is that *in extremis* I'd find myself babbling to God or down on my own knees praying to any passing deity to be granted a few more years. But I found ways, eventually, of dealing with the religious, of reconciling my agnosticism with the gratitude I felt for their prayers.

The group about which I felt no ambivalence at all was that of the committed alternativists who had researched their subject and sent me bundles of photocopied papers taken from obscure journals. They knew that orthodox medicine is a con, that unless I took control of my illness and handed it over to the naturopaths or the iridologists or whoever, then I was surely doomed.

This group all believed in the same collection of myths, prime among which was that for all its efforts orthodox medicine has not found any cure for any cancer. Four months after my diagnosis I was sitting in a barbershop in Soho where one of those day-time audience discussion shows was playing on the

TV. A woman who'd spent a small fortune on plastic surgery was defending her obsession against a member of the audience outraged at her profligate narcissism. 'Just think: you could have spent that money on cancer research,' she said, rather missing the point.

'It's a known fact,' said the surgery junkie, primly, 'that not a single life has been saved by cancer research.'

I still have the slight mark in my head where the scissors clipped me as I jumped in the barber's chair. Not a voice in the studio was raised to argue against this 'known fact', despite it being completely untrue. And yet I continue to get the letters: radiotherapy, says one correspondent, kills as many people as it cures. The death rate for most cancers, say half a dozen others, is the same now as it was in 1960/during the War/in Queen Victoria's day. If the death rate does seem to have improved then it has nothing to do with the efforts of the medical orthodoxy and everything to do with skewed statistical reporting.

The truth is that more people are cured of cancer now than ever before and more who aren't cured are helped to live longer, and often to live those extra years in some comfort.

Here's Sherwin B. Nuland, the US surgeon, teacher and writer, in *How We Die*[1]:

In the year I was born, 1930, only one in five people diagnosed with cancer survived five years. By the 1940s the figure was one in four. The effect of modern biomedicine's research capacity began to make itself felt in the 1960s, when the proportion of survivors reached one in three. At the present time 40 per cent of all cancer patients are alive five years after diagnosis; making proper statistical allowances for those who die of some unrelated cause, such as heart disease or stroke, 50 per cent survive at least that long.

1. Sherwin B. Nuland, *How We Die*, Vintage, 1998.

C

I have tried passing on that fact to some of my correspondents but invariably they skirt it. The truth is, they say, that the incidence of cancer has doubled, trebled in the past n years. Which is true enough, but doesn't have a lot to do with cure statistics or the efficacy of doctors. Cancer is more common now than it once was, but as much as anything else that's because having learned to cure or hold off so many other causes of death we live long enough to get cancer. Or they say that the only reason people live for that arbitrary five years is because detection methods are better nowadays and we're picking up cancers sufficiently early to allow people that five-year gap between detection and death. Which again would make sense were it not for the statistics which show that the number of people living longer than five years after detection is increasing too.

Invariably those who argue against orthodox medicine are waving the flag for one form of alternative medicine or another. Or, as is often the case, for more than one form of alternative medicine, for one of the striking things about alternative medicine is that if an adherent believes in one technique they'll almost certainly believe in every other technique.

Five chapters in, then, let me tell you that where I stand on alternative medicine is roughly where the Pope stands on getting drunk on the communion wine and pulling a couple of nuns.

I have, I will grant you, the journalist's luxury of self-opinionation. I know that when doctors write books on cancer they have to tread carefully when it comes to alternativism lest they offend the sensibilities of those who are happy to commune with their reflexologist once a week. I need make no such concession although to be fair to myself I'm not quite the snarling sceptic I affect to be in print. And certainly however scathing I am about the alternativists it's not because I feel the medical or pharmaceutical establishment is either so pure or so unjustly put-upon that it needs my protection.

And it's not as if I haven't tried the alternatives myself.

When I was 30 I went to my doctor complaining of the sort of non-specific symptoms you get, I now understand, when you sustain each 22-hour working, playing day with two packs of cigarettes and irregular portions of junk food. Being 30 and still nominally immortal, I was convinced there was some subtler biochemical reason for my general panicky, fluey symptoms, and that I was suffering from a specific illness. Like so many who walk hopefully into their GPs' surgeries I knew that if enough tests were carried out on me a single unified diagnosis could be made, a single pill prescribed and I would feel healthy and whole again, as was my right.

What I got instead were sleeping pills.

And then I came across a book which described my symptoms perfectly and in miraculous detail. In fact the book listed so many symptoms that I'd imagine 98 per cent of the population was covered by its thesis which, briefly described, was that civilised though we are, we have spent most of our time on Earth living in caves and eating nuts, grains and berries. Our bodies simply haven't yet had a chance to adapt to hunting and gathering in Sainsbury's.

The result, said the book, is that most of us are allergic to more foods than we can imagine including, such is the perversity of human physiology, some foods which our Neanderthal forefathers ate happily.

I was converted. I was a multiple allergic. I didn't need a pill: I needed a change of diet. I needed to eat as cavemen had eaten on rice cakes and peanut butter and eggs and honey.

C

For a few days the regime worked. Most such introspective regimes do: we all feel the better for a little guiltless self-concern. And when at the end of a couple of weeks I found I'd lapsed back into my tired and unhappy ways I blamed not the regime but my implementation of it. My problem wasn't that I was not, after all, an allergee, but that I hadn't yet discovered which foods triggered my allergies.

At the back of the book was a list of associations and societies to help the allergically challenged, one of which gave me the name of a man in West London who'd be able to help.

I'd decided to suspend my scepticism for the duration of whatever treatment he would propose, but it wasn't necessary: this man was a real scientist with a real biochemistry degree and a real white coat. For half an hour he listened to my symptoms and took long notes, and at the end of it he told me that I was almost certainly allergic to – well, *something*.

Using the old methods of sub-lingual and subcutaneous tests, he said, it could take weeks to find out the source of my allergies. But he had a new method, a method by which I could be tested for a reaction to scores of possible allergens in a single afternoon. The allergens were here in his consulting room. Lining the wall were shelves full of hundreds of little glass bottles with labels reading 'chocolate' and 'house dust mite' and 'clementine' and 'peanut butter'.

As I must know, he said, the muscles and the nerves use electricity to do their job. One of the things allergens do, he went on, is to disrupt the efficient flow of power along the body's own national grid.

'Let me,' he said, 'demonstrate.'

He made me hold out my right arm at right angles to my body.

'You can lock that arm in position, right?'

I could. He put both of his hands at my outstretched wrist and pushed downwards.

'See? I can't break the lock.'

He reached up and chose a handful of little bottles from his allergen collection. I would hold one in my left hand, he would push down on my outstretched right hand. Most of the time my arm stayed locked at the shoulder; once in a while he would be able to break the lock and my arm would be pushed down.

'You see – the allergens are interfering with the flow of electricity.'

By the end of the afternoon he was able to give me a list of the foods to which I was allergic – broccoli, tangerines, sprouts – and threw in, gratuitously I thought, a diagnosis of a candida infestation of my gut for luck.

I kept my disbelief in suspension for a while after the treatment finished, but eventually realised that I stood more chance of getting my life back if I gave up late nights and cigarettes than if I gave up Brussels sprouts and tangerines. In fact I didn't think about the allergist again until some years later when I was explaining his theories to an overworking, overplaying friend who'd been feeling panicky-fluey and who thought it might be an allergy. I told her about my man in Bayswater and my sprouts allergy.

'But how can you be sure his theory was wrong?' she said, looking worryingly hopeful. 'It may be that allergens really do interfere with electrical flow. What's this guy's number?'

I made a half-hearted attempt to stop her in her gullible tracks, but I couldn't find an absolute reason why the allergist must have been wrong.

Until it occurred to me.

The bottles containing the electricity-disrupting allergens were

C

plastic. Plastic is an insulator: electricity cannot pass through it. Not even alternative electricity.

This anecdote is, in itself, not a complete critique of alternative medicine, although I'd hold it to be a pretty substantial critique of the nature of the relationship between client and practitioner and between the two of them and the laws of physical science. My general complaint is simpler: almost every alternative diagnostic and treatment system which has ever been held up to scientific scrutiny has failed to stand up. Yes, I grant you: there have been one or two trials of homoeopathy which have suggested that there might be some effect at work here – but the trials have suggested no more than that and there have been many more which have completely failed to find any effect at all. These, oddly enough, are not the sort of odds the alternativists allow when they study the trials of orthodox medicine. A single trial in favour of one alternative regime or another out of 100 against is always enough to support it; a single trial against out of 100 in favour is always enough to damn an orthodox treatment.

Perhaps this is, as many of my correspondents tell me, a failure of science rather than of the alternatives to orthodox medicine and that science is not the right tool to determine the efficacy of iridology or aromatherapy or whatever. But this is to believe that the word 'science' describes something other than a series of usually pretty simple techniques for determining what is. A baby crawling around the floor for the first time is performing a series of scientific experiments by which she learns that floors are solid things which don't let you fall through them. Later she might learn that there are special sorts of floor which do let you fall through – woodwormy floors or paper floors – but even then there is a consistency: a floor does not behave one way when it is being studied and another when it's on its own.

And as for babies and floors, so for scientists and alternative medicine. All science has ever done with the alternative methods is to say 'Here are 100 people who are ill; here are 100 homoeopaths who say they can cure them: let's see if they get better.' All right: it's slightly more complicated than that, but the basic principle is there.

What's more, there is no reason why most alternatives should work: many of them actually conflict with what we know about the world – and by 'we' I don't just mean scientists but also those babies who have worked out the consistency of the nature of physical things. And more than that, I have objections to the way most alternative regimes came about. For while orthodox medicine has evolved gradually over the years on the basis of observation and experimentation – and yes, I know that evolution has included long and recent periods of believing the unbelievable, the untrue and the downright harmful – most alternative regimes appeared, fully formed, in the heads of their creators. They were guesses or hunches converted overnight into fixed principles and...

But see? You've gone and got me started now.

The bottom line, as far as I can see, is this. Homoeopathy has been going since the mid-nineteenth century, naturopathy for some hundreds of years in various forms; reflexology is based on principles and charts which pre-date most orthodox medical principles. Much the same goes for herbalism, iridology, acupuncture and any of the medical systems emanating from the traditions of the mystic East.

One of the principles which is common to most of these systems is that they have hardly changed from the day of their inception; indeed many of their adherents take pride in the immutability of their principles.

And yet until the early part of this century the percentage of cancer victims cured of their illness had remained more or less the same since the year dot. Enter nasty orthodox medicine, self-serving, arrogant, ignorant of lines of energy and pressure points, focused on the symptom rather than the whole person, and what do you know? Suddenly people start recovering from cancer.

For all this, though, I can see the temptation of going the alternative route. At the Marsden I'd more or less given up any personal control of my illness. Here I was diagnosed as having a cancer which had originated no one knew where, a cancer which had a chance of killing me, and I was allowing people I'd never met to prod me and poke me and slice me up and subject me to dangerous rays following principles I didn't quite understand.

How much better it would be if I could do something for myself, something based on some simple and obvious principle – that energy lines connect different parts of the body, that you are what you eat, that biochemical equilibrium can be reached by scourging the toxins from your skin – which would allow me to take control of my cancer. How wonderful it would be to decide for myself which of the dozens of equally valid remedies from around the world was most suitable for my personality, my cancer, my birth sign.

I couldn't do it, though. I went for radiotherapy instead.

My porno-mask and the results of my simulation had been sent down to the Varian suite. The notes showed a map of the cross-section of my head and neck with, on the left-hand side of my neck, an irregular round-edged shape some few inches long marked as the mass of the tumour. In reality the shape represented no more than the furthest extent of where Henk thought a primary site might be and the area at which the radiation would be fired for the next six weeks.

Life for those six weeks became the nearest I've had to a daily routine since I gave up going into an office in the early 80s. And quite quickly the Varian suite became as mundane as any office and I found myself considering how the exciting and the terrifying can become transformed equally by familiarity into the banal and the boring. At 14, when puberty hadn't yet kicked in completely with its full complement of benisons, I ached to reach an age where I needed to shave daily; by 18 I'd happily have had the beard removed by electrolysis for the chance of an extra ten minutes' kip each morning. Whatever the circumstance, ordinariness inevitably reasserts itself and there is no human activity which can't have the wind knocked out of it by being converted into a routine.

This was my new routine:

At 3.30 each day I'd drive the couple of miles or so to the hospital.

At 4.05 I'd announce my arrival by sticking my appointment card into the upper of the two clips on the wall of the radiotherapy suite's waiting room, the one for the slightly less clever of the two radiology machines.

From 4.06 to 4.10 I'd flip through the property pages of one of the copies of *Country Life* left lying about the waiting room and live the brief metropolitan daydream of the pound-for-pound conversion of a medium-sized city home into a mansion standing in 25 acres of somewhere cold and inaccessible.

At 4.10 a radiologist would call my name and I'd stroll into the barn-sized room with its irradiating machine in the middle of it. One of the three radiologists would offer a cheery 'How are you

C

then?' and I'd say 'Well, since you ask, I've got cancer' and it is a tribute to their saintliness that even those radiologists who'd heard this tired gag six or seven times never smacked me in my irradiated teeth.

At 4.13 I'd strip to the waist and bemoan my lost weight, of which more later. Suffice to say, for the time being, that on the day of my diagnosis I weighed something like $14^1/2$ stone and as I write some six months later I've dropped to just under 10 stone although this first course of radiotherapy cost me no more than two or three stone. As far as I was concerned, the weight loss had nothing to do with the cancer eating away at my corporation but was because the various biopsies and lump removals meant that for much of the month preceding the radiotherapy I'd not been able to eat. I was wrong: it was to do with the cancer.

At 4.15 I'd lie down on the machine's bench and the radiographer would clamp my mask over my face and upper chest, pressing the back of my head on to a padded metal plate. Had you told me a month earlier that I would spend 15 minutes a day thus constrained I'd have told you about my small claustrophobia problem and tried not to vomit in your lap at the thought. But even claustrophobia becomes routine.

I'd be millimetrically aligned under the green laser beam set into the ceiling and a button would be pressed. I'd count the warning beeper's 53 beeps (46 if the small machine was being serviced and I was laid out on the big one next door), the nine seconds' silence, the 29 seconds' buzzing while the machine irradiated away to itself. The warning beeps are to give the radiologists time to get out of the room and behind the lead screening. They know, as do the alternativists, that radiation is dangerous stuff reserved for atom bomb victims and cancer patients.

The radiologists would return, realign the machine, press the button, 53 beeps, nine seconds' silence, 29 seconds' buzzing, and then twice more again.

I was, I thought, being cured.

Chapter 6

I once had two or three sessions, but no more than that, with a rather up-market hypnotherapist – a man with a winter tan and a professionally sincere smile and cuff-linked shirt-sleeves, who laid me on a leather couch and smooth-talked me to semi-sleep. Nominally the idea was to cure me of smoking but he was one of those holistic types who deal with the whole psyche and he said that while he was in there he might as well roll up his sleeves and tweak a few other dangerous neuroses.

Hypnotherapy turned out to be a jokey collusion between therapist and therapee in which he would pretend to put me under the influence and I would pretend to have transcended to a sort of lumber room of the psyche wherein were all sorts of old thoughts and fears and childhood events lying about on the floor waiting for me to inspect them. Three or four times a session I'd pick up one of these items and wave it around for the therapist to look at, although the reason I stopped was because he kept on goading me to try and find some event or other which would induce a useful bit of screaming and a panic attack.

After he'd brought me round we'd talk about what we'd found in the room, both of us pretending that we'd discovered a place that I had no idea existed. In fact, as he must have known, it was a place I knew full well was there, and I knew most of its contents too. It was like the loft of my house: not a space I'd ever think to list in an inventory of rooms and containing all sorts of useless junk, but a room, nonetheless, which never came as a surprise to me.

One of the things at which I clutched and of which we were both terribly proud was the discovery of the first time I thought of myself as overweight. Not fat, you understand, because heavy as I've been I've never had the fat boy's take on life or worn the fat boy's clothes or walked his waddling walk. I was, rather, a boy and then a man destined to spend his life asking the shop assistant if they had it in L, and while they were there they might as well bring the XL too, just in case.

Anyway, I recalled that the first time I had a real sense of this I must have been eight or nine, and sitting on a low wall in my grandmother's garden in Hackney. It was summer and I was in bathing trunks. And to please the hypnotherapist I allowed myself to discover the memory of my mother pointing at the tiny roll of puppy fat at the bend in my stomach, and myself looking down at it and knowing it shouldn't be there.

All of which sounds a terribly *Mommy Dearest* sort of moment, but wasn't at all. Indeed, if it had been more than a passing fond comment on Mum's part I might not have been $14\frac{1}{2}$ stone on the day I was diagnosed cancerous. I might have been my actuarially ideal weight of 12 stone – less than I weighed, in fact, when the hospital started worrying about my weight loss.

Losing weight was one of the phenomena which entered my cancer joke book pretty quickly. 'Hey – have you lost weight?' acquaintances who didn't know the deal would say.

'A bit actually, yes,' I'd say proudly, as if I'd been working hard at it, and then:

'Cancer. It's a great diet,' and wait for the reaction. In truth, once I'd found a more sensitive way of sharing the news it exited my joke book just as quickly as it had arrived.

Not that I'd found a way of dealing with the explanation which worked every time. Our social life had, by this time, shrunk somewhat – in part because we were both tired and in part because our priorities had changed and suddenly turning up to celebrate the publishing of a book we wouldn't read by an author we barely knew seemed a less than positive way to fill an evening. We'd stopped giving dinner parties more or less, and rarely went to them, but there was one we'd accepted before radiotherapy started and which was suddenly upon us, and we thought it was about time we got out.

Imagine: you turn up at a dinner party with a dozen people and there in the middle of the long side of the table is a bloke you've never met before, and he's not eating. It's not that he's not eating in the way that humourless vegetarians don't eat, or in the manner of those stick-thin women who say 'That was *delicious* and I'm so *full*' in the hope that if they gush enough you won't notice they sucked briefly on a couple of beans and hid a shitake mushroom under their fork.

No: he's not eating as if this simply isn't an eating occasion, as if nobody told him that food would be served. There is a plate, but it is empty, and cutlery too, but it is untouched.

Well, you'd say something, wouldn't you?

'Can I pass you anything?' said a woman as if she wasn't sure whether I'd noticed the food piled up along the table. 'What would you like?' said another, hesitantly, as if I might be subject to delusions and expect to be fed off gold plate.

'Nothing, thanks.' I grinned as if not eating were one of the usual options at dinner parties. What could I say? Egocentrically, it hadn't occurred to me that people wouldn't know, and you can't just smile and say 'No, nothing for me: I've got cancer', can you? It is both too much of an explanation and not enough of one. It stops conversations, begs questions to which the asker really doesn't want to hear the answer, demands a too carefully crafted response.

And so I did the worst, and rudest, thing of all. Eventually somebody said 'I wish I could lose weight that way' and I said, truculently, 'You would do if you had cancer too', except that I compounded the rudeness by muttering it so that some of the

C

table heard nothing and the rest thought they'd picked up on some sort of tasteless joke.

It screwed up the dinner party for the best part of an hour and induced a lot of piercing glowers from Nigella on the other side of the table, and I sat in silence thinking of a couple of dozen ways in which I could have handled it better.

It was the radiotherapy that did it. The principle of gradual disclosure had prepared me for those things which the radiation would almost certainly do to me – no saliva, sore throat, the odd missing tuft of hair – but not for many of the things it only *might* do. In fact the saliva stayed and the throat was never that sore, albeit that it still hurt pretty badly after the biopsy, but nobody thought to tell me about the effect on my taste-buds. At least now that I come to think of it they may have mentioned that I'd lose the use of my taste-buds, but they said nothing about the devastation that eventuality would wreak on my emotional and corporeal equilibrium.

There is, I remember from the days when I thought the metaphysical poets had greater insights into the teenage mind even than Jethro Tull or the Doors, a sermon written by John Donne wearing his deanery hat in which he praises God for all his works and in particular for that work which causes the raddled nose of the tertiary syphilitic to drop off. That way, said Donne, the dying wretch avoids smelling his own putrefying flesh.

And that, I think, is the last time God attached a pure thought to a nasty disease. Once He'd done syphilis He determined that the side-effect of any given illness would be nastier than the illness itself and that the metaphorical ingrowing toenail would never numb the metaphorical foot to make the metaphorical hike more pleasurable. And as for illness, so for the treatment of illness, for surely there can be no intrinsic reason why the side-effects of any given medical regime should be even nastier than the complaint it treats, why a barium meal shouldn't taste like a steak dinner or why a tourniquet shouldn't lead to a pleasant tingling sensation rather than to gangrene. Specifically, in my case, why can't the side-effect of radiotherapy be to make therapees ravenously hungry and super-sensitive to mother nature's bounteous tastes in a way that would actually speed recovery? Would it be too much to ask that just once physics and human biology co-operate in some fortuitous way that made us slightly giggly, light-headed creatures rather than mild depressives? No wonder the alternative quacks get away with their fairy dust treatments: you die just as quickly as with the real thing but you feel better about it.

Two weeks into the treatment, with my throat buzzing with radioactivity, I felt for the first time as if I had cancer. People would say, in that reverential chapel-of-rest voice, 'How *are* you?' and assume the list of symptoms I'd reel off were those of cancer. They weren't: they were the symptoms of being cured of cancer, of the surgical excavations in my throat and of the radiotherapy. And, as the nature-never-compensates thesis dictates, the curative symptoms were the last ones I needed.

In the bathroom and beside my bed the evidence of disease was piling up. There were the industrial strength, prescription-only painkillers to cope with the pain from the biopsy: the giant bottle of co-dydramol, the economy-sized box of co-codamol, the blister sheets of Voltarol. There was the anti-emetic to counter the nausea that the radiotherapy had started to induce, and the fluoride gel to spread over my gums, and the sleeping pills to help me forget about all the other pills I was taking.

But worse than the pain, worse than having to take the

indigestion-stirring, constipating cures for the pain, was the loss of the sense of taste.

In truth, I was surprised the loss was as depressing as it turned out to be. I've always prided myself in a sly sort of way of being the king of the Spam fritter, the man whom the avocado revolution entirely passed by in the 70s and who managed to get all the way through the late 80s without eating a sun-dried tomato. If you'd asked my pre-cancerous self which of its senses it could most afford to lose it would almost certainly have gone for taste. If you'd asked the wife of my pre-cancerous self – a woman who is, *inter alia*, the food writer at *Vogue*, wrote a restaurant column for a dozen years, and can turn any three ingredients into a sublime feast – she'd have told you that I was a food-philistine, a man who'd never miss his taste-buds because, as far as she was aware, he'd never had any.

Perhaps it wouldn't have been so bad if my complete complement of taste-buds had been entirely pulverised by the rays, but a few held on, still twitching slightly in their agony, and making sure that the very slight memory of taste which filtered through was, uniformly and regardless of what I tried to eat, nauseating. Worse: I still had a memory of what tastes had been like so recently, and a sense of smell, and thus was surprised, and depressed, anew every time I ate something to discover that it tasted of rancid wallpaper paste.

Each day I would find myself remembering a taste – peanut butter, banana bread, cornflakes in cold milk – and recalling it so vividly that I became convinced that this taste would still be accessible to me. And so I'd lather a slice of bread with peanut butter, or fill a bowl with cornflakes, or ask Nigella to run up some banana bread, and I'd take a deep breath, close my eyes, fill my mouth in the absolute conviction that this time I'd have found something that transcended my new disability, something on which I could subsist until the buds returned in a month or four. And each time I'd find myself spitting out another mouthful of inedible poison. Eventually even the rancid wallpaper taste disappeared as everything – water included – took on the taste of battery acid.

It was depressing and at the same time infuriating, and I started reacting to the regular rediscovery of my crocked mouth with a rage which I'd been told would accompany the original diagnosis ('some patients find they are *angry* with their cancer' was the sort of thing the books said) but hadn't. I hurled the food, thumped the table, stormed out of the room, shouted at Nigella, avoided the children lest I take it out on them. And then ten minutes later I'd be back, remorseful, apologetic like some cheesy drunk promising never to touch another drop. I didn't react this way every time, but I did it often enough to scare myself and worry Nigella.

By the fourth week of radiotherapy I was on a diet which consisted entirely of Ready-Brek – a sort of cowardly porridge – and poached egg on toast. I was losing weight fast.

Although I wasn't to hit my lowest weight for another few months, I was already running out of wardrobe. Luckily I was at the Marsden every day – a hospital within 500 yards of some dozens of clothes shops in Fulham and Chelsea. Early on in the illness I'd discovered that as a cancer patient I had an advantage over other men. I was meeting Bywater at a Soho club for lunch and passed a shop selling £400 leather jackets for a knock-down £299. I bought one. I was, I thought, entitled. I had cancer, for Christ's sake. What sort of world was this where a man with cancer couldn't buy himself a leather jacket? I arrived home that afternoon wearing the jacket and with one of the standard stories

C

prepared – I'd spilled something on the jacket I'd been wearing; it had suddenly turned cold; the jacket was only £199, or £99. But it wasn't necessary. Nigella thought I was entitled too. From where she was standing, bless her, if a leather jacket cheered me up then never mind the American Express bill that hadn't yet been paid.

The principle extended to my new wardrobe. It was bad enough, we decided, that I had cancer without having to have cancer *and* be dressed in clothes two sizes too big. And, what the hell, we could pay the Amex bill next month.

And so once or twice a week I'd rise from the radiotherapy bench and dress and we'd walk down to one of the shops along the road and cheer me up with a new suit or a new pair of trousers or a new sweater in my new size. Sometimes we didn't even wait for a radiotherapy day in Fulham; one Sunday I did so much damage in Selfridge's various departments that the Visa people phoned the cash desk after my card had been swiped to check whether it was really me because I was spending at the rate usually seen only in those who have stolen a credit card and are getting the best use out of it before the loss is reported.

Eventually I realised there was a subtler reason behind all this spending which involved another appeal to the hubris gods. After all, if I could get into deep enough money trouble they'd have to keep me alive so that I could suffer those consequences. Alternatively when the gods looked down they would see a humble, if astonishingly well dressed, man unwilling to make the assumption that he'd put back any of the weight he'd lost, which is to say unwilling to assume that he'd get better. Impressed by this humility, they would allow him to get better, not least so that he could rue his expensive new wardrobe full of tiny and unwearable clothes.

But if the weight loss was doing wonders for my wardrobe it was worrying the medical team. Or, rather, my growing medical team, for I had acquired, in addition to my surgeon and doctor and radiotherapist and radiologist and dentist, a dietitian.

The job of the modern dietitian is pretty easy and consists, for the most part, in telling people to stop eating anything enjoyable and start eating bean sprouts. Cancer dietitians, though, live in a nutritional dystopia where everything which medical science has spent the last 25 years proving is bad, is deemed good.

Remember how things were in the pre-cholesterol era? How your mother would look at your plate at the end of a meal and say 'But you've left the best bit!' with 'best' meaning 'most wholesome', and how the best bit always turned out to be precisely the thing – bacon rind, the fatty stump of a chop, the thick cream at the top of a glass of milk – which doctors later discovered you should never eat? Those are precisely the bits the nutritionist would recommend. After a session with her Nigella would comb the supermarket shelves for anything that was four parts lard, or half sugar, and that could be whizzed up into a semi-solid paste and swallowed before the crippled taste-buds noticed it was there.

Indeed, there were whole areas of the disease and the treatment which Nigella had taken over from me and from the doctors. It was Nigella who made the calls to fix the various appointments, Nigella who spent time talking to editors and producers, cancelling shows and rearranging deadlines, Nigella who cooked special meals I fancied on some whim or another and who commiserated when I could only eat a mouthful, Nigella who got up for the children and who coped when a few months into all of this our nanny resigned, Nigella who lay with me at night and talked about what was happening and made some of

C

the fear and the frustration go away.

It was Nigella too who reassured me about my professional life.

For the first few weeks of treatment nothing much had changed with my work. The *Times* column had become a cancer column, although at this point not exclusively so, and I had no real problem keeping up with my other regular gigs writing about the media for the *Evening Standard* and reviewing TV for the *New Statesman*. Radio, though, was becoming a problem.

I had two regular programmes on BBC radio: *After Hours*, a late night live, two-hour talk show on Radio 5 Live which involved me guiding four or five professional gabblers through a single subject each week, and *Fourth Column* on Radio 4 which had me presenting four columnar wits to the microphone every Friday night. I loved doing both shows and was proud, in my insecure 'Look, Ma – top of the world' way to have the jobs. Dr Henk had made it clear at our first meeting that as far as he was concerned radiotherapy rendered all broadcasting an impossibility: my voice would be too croaky, my throat too painful and I'd be too tired. On that basis I dropped *After Hours* almost immediately radiotherapy started: even I understood that two hours' live chat was probably beyond me.

Fourth Column was a different matter. While *After Hours* was long, unscripted and live, and demanded that, *in extremis*, I could be called upon to keep the talk going under my own steam, *Fourth Column* was short, scripted and recorded. Indeed, although it was nominally my programme and appeared under my name in the *Radio Times*, I usually had no more than five or six minutes of script to write and read each week. I told Brian King, its long-standing producer, what the problem was and said that I'd like to try and keep the job going on the understanding that there might come a time when my voice just couldn't cope and somebody else would have to step in. It was a suggestion which I didn't expect King to agree to for a moment; why, after all, should the BBC's output suffer for my throat? To my amazement, and delight, he agreed to the proposal as if it were the most normal thing in the world.

To my greater amazement he kept me going through the whole of the next two series, even though at one point the radiotherapy gave me the rasping voice of a bottle-a-day alcoholic combined with a new lisp brought on by the collapse of one of my lingual nerves under the combined pressure of the biopsy and the radiation.

Generally speaking, though, I decided to turn down most other broadcasting until after the radiotherapy was over and my throat had healed. The one exception was just after the May 1st election when *Newsnight* phoned up and asked me to come on and talk to Jeremy Paxman about the recently disgraced ex-MP Neil Hamilton who was appearing that night with his wife Christine on *Have I Got News For You*. It was the sort of ten-minute punditry that is bread and butter for freelance mouths like mine and for some reason I decided that I needed to prove to myself that I could still talk to a camera.

As it happened that day I'd acquired a new pharmaceutical toy: a large plastic syringe full of local anaesthetic gel. The radiotherapy had, understandably enough, caused one side of my mouth to break out in giant ulcers which not only further affected my ability to eat but also meant I had to be careful with my speech. The gel lasted for minutes before it was washed away by my saliva and so I was leaving its application until just before the camera went on me.

I'd met Jeremy Paxman just a few times at various Notting Hill parties and although there was no reason why he should have

C

known about my cancer, I assumed without much thinking about it that because most of the West London media lot seemed to know about it so would he. I was slipped into my pundit's chair while the previous item was running, two minutes before I was due to give the word on Hamilton. Paxman was flipping through his script and looked up to say hello. He saw me apparently injecting something into my gums.

'What's that for? Broadcast nerves?' he said, and laughed.

I gave the stupidest answer, all things considered.

'Er, no. Throat cancer.'

'Seriously?'

'Well, yes. I'm sorry, I thought they'd—'

At which point the green light went and we were on air. Say what you like about Paxman, but the man's a professional. Looking back at a tape of the interview there are only two moments where the pauses are long enough to suggest that his interviewee has just announced he's got cancer.

I gave up TV for a while after that and decided that I simply wouldn't do it again until the radiotherapy was over, my voice had returned, the swelling around my operation scar had disappeared and I'd been given the all clear which I would certainly get given the 92 per cent cure rate of my sort of cancer.

And I would have got it too, had they not discovered the primary.

Chapter 7

C

If the statistics were anything to go by then the final radiotherapy session should have marked my last officially cancerous day. It felt more like my first. Towards the end of the treatment I'd had problems: the back of my neck was so badly burned by the third of the four daily bursts of radiation that Henk had ordered that pass of the ray gun to be discontinued a week or so before the final session. But even reducing my dose didn't help my general feelings of wretchedness and, like a prisoner who makes a jail-break when his sentence is almost over, I found that which had been bearable suddenly all seemed too much. I seriously considered not turning up for treatment on the last few days. If 30 sessions of radiotherapy can fix me, I told one of the radiotherapists, then so can 27 or 28. But no: the deal is that such is the power of radiation that they give the minimum necessary to treat the cancer. Any more and there's a chance that the cure will be nastier than the illness – or even induce further cancers; any less and it simply might not be enough to do the job.

And so I staggered along, tired, thin, dispirited, with no real sense that anything was coming to an end.

I seemed to have lost that trick I'd developed early on of affecting to be cool about cancer. What's more, although I'd started the treatment by congratulating myself on my well-balanced – hah! – take on my illness, I now began to feel that it really had been no more than a trick, which is to say that I'd been tricked along with everyone else.

From the start I'd worked out that I had a choice: either I could do the standard 'I'd love to but' – catch in throat – 'I've got cancer' routine which wouldn't make me feel much better and would, I thought, give everyone else a good excuse for ignoring me, or I could be relaxed about it. Relaxation, I realised, was the only choice and not least because even were I not relaxed there

C

was no way in which I could communicate my agitation on a full-time basis.

When people ask how you are you can say 'scared' but you can't *be* scared, you can't *do* scaredness for more than a moment or two. I imagine that conscripts in fox-holes waiting for mortars to drop manage to keep scaredness going for hours at a time – shivering, crying, moaning, whatever it is that the truly and continuously scared do in the hope that their scaredness will leak away from them. But I had no sense of how to be scared in any but an abstract and internal way; perhaps if I'd developed such a sense I wouldn't have been feeling so low now.

And so when readers and friends wrote to me to say how clever (or brave or sensible) it was to face my cancer with a wry smile playing about my boyish lips I affected not to know what they were talking about. When they told me that I didn't understand how courageous I was to come into the open with the details of my cancer, my eyes would go wide and I'd tell them that it hadn't occurred to me that I had any alternative. During the early part of the summer we turned up at any number of parties where people I knew only vaguely would walk across the room, lay a hand on my shoulder, look deeply into my eyes and say 'You are so...' and then add one or other from the limited menu of fortitudinous adjectives.

It was, as far as I was concerned, all bollocks. Writing about my cancer wasn't brave. Not writing about it, now that *would* have been brave. Writing the old domestic pieces about babies and Sainsbury's and being on the sharp end of feminism, and not mentioning that all these things needed to be viewed against the backdrop of the slipping chances of my being around to draw the benefits of my Spend and Save card, might have taken some courage.

What I was doing instead was looking for a way to make my cancer acceptable, to be the man who'd discovered chic cancer. I wasn't doing this for the greater good of cancer patients everywhere, for all that cancer patients everywhere wrote to thank me for the favour. I was doing it as a form of very public denial therapy. By writing about the cancer each week (and subsequently by writing this book and sitting in front of the BBC's documentary cameras) I was trying to change the problem from one of pain and physical constraint and possibly impending death into one of best journalistic practice. Faced with a new symptom, a new oncological possibility, I'd found a way of thinking of it not in terms of how it would affect my life, my psyche, my family, but of how best to share it with the readers, of how to make a momentary thought a greater philosophical reflection. And in doing so I wasn't, of course, unconscious of the times when I was putting a jaunty spin on something depressing, of the times when I was feigning bravery or indifference.

But in those last few days of radiotherapy I seemed to have lost that trick. The columns I wrote in those weeks had become either maudlin or mawkish, self-pitying or depressive. I'd had enough of all this. I couldn't be clever about it any more; I couldn't pretend cancer in the right hands was a chic and temporary accessory, not least because the cancer which was meant to have disappeared on the last day of radiotherapy, felt as if it were still around.

And, of course, as long as I believed the cancer was still in me I also believed that I was bucking the statistics – that I wasn't going to be one of the 92 per cent who was cured but one of the 8 per cent who died.

What was remarkable was the extent to which that possible

C

death remained an unspoken fear. Hardly any of the thousands who had written and would write to me about my presumed courage under cytological fire actually came clean with the details of what they thought I was being courageous about. If they were at all specific it was to say that I was brave to suffer the pain, or the depression, or the therapy. What they meant, and what I was repressing by turning the illness into a literary exercise, was that I was brave not to break down, having been told that I might soon die.

The maudlin moment passed, after a fashion. At the end of the month we had our postponed annual midsummer's party of 400 people crammed into our back garden, and that night, slim and in a shiny new suit, I felt entitled to look forward to next year's party and the one after that. But still, I didn't feel what you'd call *better*.

In fact I had only one symptom and that was the one which I'd had since the first day: I was still coughing up food. Indeed, as the radiotherapy had roughened my throat the single symptom had got worse and part of the reason I was eating so little was that every meal set me off on a painful coughing jag. Attached to the pain from the coughing was an earache – a pain which since childhood I've found more depressing than any other.

I'd told Dr Henk about the coughing and the earache at our weekly meetings, and when we met in his little cubicle a couple of days after our last session I told him about it again. It felt, I said, as if I had a lesion right at the base of my tongue, or some sort of extra flap which food was hiding behind.

Henk looked through my notes and granted that in fact I'd mentioned the problem fairly regularly, as if to suggest that he understood that I wasn't inventing the symptom. Perhaps, he said, a surgeon should take a look at it, and for 'look' read 'knife'.

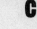

Even if Henk was now the doctor with primary charge of my illness, my surgeon was still nominally Mr Mady of Harley Street and St George's. But although Henk visited St George's to dispense radiotherapeutic wisdom, Mady wasn't a Marsden surgeon. I could, I suppose, have gone back to St George's, but the thought filled me with gloom. Most thoughts at the time filled me with gloom, it's true, but the trek through the South London suburbs was a particularly dispiriting prospect.

Nigella pressed the issue with Henk: was there not somebody at the Marsden who could do the job? Yes: the Marsden had its own head and neck surgeon, a man who specialised not just in head and neck but in cancers of the head and neck. Peter Rhŷs Evans was, like Henk, *sui generis*, he was the *ne plus ultra*, he was the man. Getting him to be my man, though, was a diplomatic exercise on a par with settling the Northern Ireland problem. Rhŷs Evans couldn't take me on without my being referred to him by a doctor. Henk couldn't refer me because I'd come to him in the first place courtesy of Mady. Mady could refer me, I imagine, but given that we didn't want to continue with him for entirely selfish reasons I wasn't going to ask him to. In the end I had to go back to my own GP, Dr Mulligan, and get him to write a letter asking Rhŷs Evans to see me as if it was Mulligan's own idea.

When Nigella and I turned up at Rhŷs Evans' Harley Street rooms (on the first floor this time: the lower the grander, I'd been told) he really did look the part of the Head and Neck Man Whose Name Is Spoken With Awe. The wall of his secretary's office was plastered with certificates from Paris and New York and South Africa as well as London: here was a man who had travelled the globe to study head and neck tumours in all their worldly variety, who had been accorded the freedom of those

C

cities where they take head and neck cancer seriously, been granted fellowships of the most prestigious Royal Colleges of Neck and International Societies of Head.

He was also, it turned out, one of the most charming of surgeons, a stocky and dapper man who looked ten years younger than his 48 years, the son of an expatriate Welsh ENT man and one who kept an aging Jaguar sports car with his initials on the number plate – the plate a present from a grateful patient – parked outside the shop.

Again I told my story from scratch while Rhŷs Evans sat behind his leather-topped not-a-doctor's desk and took longhand notes. The glandular fever, the swelling, the scan and the bloodtest and the aspiration, the cystectomy, the surprise diagnosis, the biopsy and so all the way through to a precise description of the single coughing symptom. Again, as with Mr Hinton those few months ago, the act of cataloguing the events gave them an increased meaning – doubly so since with Hinton I was still, as far as we were all concerned, cancer-free.

Rhŷs Evans walked me across to the other side of the not-a-doctor's-consulting-room and sat me in what looked like an old-fashioned barber's chair but which turned out to be the ENT chair which had been passed down from one ENT man to another over the decades since the first ENT man had taken the rooms in the 20s.

For the dozenth time I watched as a doctor warmed the nickel-plated tongue depressor on the little gas burner, for the dozenth time I opened my mouth to let a doctor look for a cancer in it, for the dozenth time I 'aahhhed' to demonstrate whether a tumour was clinging to my vocal cords. For the third time I gagged as a local anaesthetic was sprayed on the back of my throat and down one nostril, and then watched the TV monitor as the naso-endoscope was passed into my gullet.

It showed, said Rhŷs Evans, nothing at all. Certainly it didn't show whatever it was that was causing the food to return whence it came. Rhŷs Evans sent me back to the Marsden for more tests: another CT scan, some more blood tests, an X-ray, something called a barium swallow which was, I imagined, slightly less than a barium meal and possibly more than a barium snack.

A few days later I was having lunch with Georgina Henry and Roger Alton, respectively the deputy and features editors of the *Guardian*, who were grilling me about my health. Half way through the soup course Alton asked the bottom-line question: did I still have cancer? Before I could shrug my shoulders my mobile rang: it was Nigella. Rhŷs Evans had phoned. The scan seemed to show some slight swelling around the site of the defunct tonsils. The good news was that there seemed to be no enlargement of the lymph glands.

I clicked the phone off. Yes, Roger. It looked as if I still had cancer.

Well, perhaps it was a bit of an exaggeration, and obviously I was back on my ten-cool-ways-to-have-cancer routine, but certainly something was still not right. Rhŷs Evans wanted me to have another biopsy as soon as the post-radiation swelling in my throat had subsided. Nobody was saying it, but everyone was proceeding as if there was still work for them to do.

A week later Nigella and I took a cab to the Lister Hospital, a private hotel with attached operating facilities by the Thames at Chelsea. As we moved through the West London traffic we tried to divine what the biopsy would show. There was, after all, no obvious sign of a cancer, no bleeding or ulceration or swelling. As the traffic jammed in the King's Road I idly poked a finger into my mouth and towards the area at the back of my throat where the food seemed to be getting trapped.

'Christ! I can feel a lump,' I said to Nigella.

'What sort of lump?' she asked, sounding as panicky as I suddenly felt.

'A sort of... hold on. No: it's a bit of gum.'

I had, for some inexplicable reason, started chewing the occasional nicotine chewing gum again. At first it was squares of gum which were left over from my pre-cancerous days and which I'd found hibernating in odd drawers or jacket pockets, but a couple of days before I'd actually bought a pack of the things. I remembered Keith Castle, the first successful British heart transplant patient, who even that close to death couldn't bring himself to give up smoking. Perhaps if he'd had gum to chew he'd be alive still. Perhaps, like me, he'd find that little bits of gum detached themselves and got stuck in balls around the mouth and throat.

I prodded again.

'No... hold on. Shit. It *is* a lump.'

It was, too: a small thickening of the skin at the very base of my tongue, rather as if the thing had become calloused from too much talking.

The panic of this new discovery aside, the Lister with its pretend-grand institutional fittings and its air-hostess nurses' uniforms was, if anything, slightly more depressing than St George's, but Nigella and I lay on my hospital bed and watched afternoon TV and forgot, for a moment, why we were there. Halfway through *Quincy* an air-hostess nurse came in to take my blood pressure and I wondered why private hospitals go for the modern look with their nurses. If I were paying out my own money, rather than BUPA's, I'd want to see nurses dressed in precisely the reassuring old-fashioned starched creations that the NHS has dropped.

'Do you want your girlfriend to stay?' she said.

'My wife,' I said.

'Oh, right. It's just that you looked so happy together that I thought, you know...' Who knows: this might be a piece of standard private-medicine flummery, but it cheered me up no end.

As *Perry Mason* started Rhŷs Evans came to see me. How was I? Were there any changes? Any new symptoms?

Nothing really, I told him. Just this slight hardness right at the back of my mouth near where my tongue is. Rhŷs Evans gave it a surgical prod and shrugged. He'd have a look in a minute.

They wheeled me down to the surgery and Nigella stayed to watch the end of *Perry Mason*. I was home that night with a new bottle of painkillers to numb the effects of having more slivers of throat removed.

My diary for that week in the middle of July shows a period in limbo: a poker evening, a drink with an editor, a couple of work meetings, some lunches, two parties. I'd started back at *After Hours* again, and managed to cram a couple of editions in. Abnormal as my life felt at the time, it turned out to be my last week of normality. In the diary the usual gallivanting continues into the next week, the only difference being that the meetings and the parties and the drinks all have cancelling lines struck through them. Above them, in tiny letters to fit the reduced space, are entries naming new names, new characters in my about-to-be-new life: Jemima Harrison, Olivia Lichtenstein, Nicholas Breach, Stephanie Kingham.

We met Peter Rhŷs Evans again in his rooms. The hardness at the base of my tongue had indeed been cancer. Now I had a

C

specific cancer: not just cancer of the neck and head, but cancer of the tongue, a particular sort of cancer with particular characteristics. As far as he could tell it was about an inch or so in diameter and he would have to cut it out. At the same time he would have to work on my neck. We knew that the cancer in the cyst and that in the lymph node next to it were secondaries: he needed to know how far along my lymphatic system the cancer had travelled. He intended taking out the dozen or so lymph glands on both sides of my neck in the hope that there would be two pairs free of any cancer, showing the furthest extent of the disease. If all the glands on either side were cancerous he'd know, he implied, that the probability was that the cancer had spread beyond my neck.

How did I feel? Neutral, I suppose. Nothing Rhŷs Evans said came as much of a surprise. I knew I had cancer and I knew in my waters that the cancer hadn't been chased off by the radiotherapy. Overwhelming sympathy and anxiety aside, Nigella felt a mixture of self-recrimination and anger. Just before the radiotherapy had started we'd mentioned the coughing and the earache to Henk's registrar. He'd said that if we liked the hospital could arrange a proper endoscopy – the sort which involved a general anaesthetic. The only trouble was, he said, that we'd have to postpone radiotherapy for a week. I wanted to get the therapy over with as soon as possible; Nigella didn't push the point. Now she felt that had she done so they might have found the tumour a couple of months earlier. It's unlikely that the two months would have made a difference to the spread of a cancer which must have been around for years, but it would almost certainly have made a difference to the original treatment.

Rhŷs Evans is an optimist with an optimist's infectious good cheer and so we left him with the sustaining thought that at last the doctors had found something they could doctor rather than that I was about to undergo a big-deal operation. But there was that principle of gradual disclosure at work again. It turned out that my secondaries are pretty often the result of tongue cancers and that the earache was a common symptom. Nobody, of course, had mentioned this before.

Bywater came round that night and went into upbeat mode again. This was *great* news, he said. They had found the primary, they would cut it out, in a year's time I would have forgotten I ever had cancer. Perhaps he should have been a doctor, after all. As with the other doctors there was no mention of the fact that it had been equally great news when they *hadn't* been able to find a primary site because that meant it was so small that it could be zapped by the radiotherapy.

But I felt pretty sanguine about the whole thing. I imagined a fairly routine operation to cut a bit out of me, stitch me up and kick me out on to the street again.

I phoned up Jemima Harrison and told her the news. Harrison was a journalist then working as an assistant producer in the BBC documentaries department under Olivia Lichtenstein, the editor of the *Inside Story* series. I'd met Harrison on, of all uncool places, the Internet some weeks before. She had been charged to work up some programme ideas for the department and we were discussing a number together, including one for a series about cancer. Lichtenstein had known Nigella from one or other of their previous incarnations and our daughters went to the same Saturday morning ballet classes.

I'd told Harrison that it looked as if my own cancer story wasn't yet over. She talked to Lichtenstein and they decided to start work on the cancer programme/series/whatever there and then without a formal proposal or really any idea what sort of televisual event we were talking about. Instead of being about cancer generally it would be about my cancer – which wasn't quite what I had in mind. I had seen myself presenting the sort of thing the *Radio Times* lists as 'A Major New Series on Disease Which Affects One Briton in Three' full of carefully scripted walking-talking pieces to camera and clever graphics showing cancer cells invading major organs; they seemed to see a frowning man in pyjamas candidly voicing his fears to a close-up lens. We could, I thought, argue the toss when this was all over – whenever that would now be. Meanwhile it meant the that next time we met Rhŷs Evans it was with the cameras running.

This time, and with a couple of days to go, he took us through the operation. It would, he said, take around six hours. He would dissect my neck, sending the glands down to the histopathology labs as he removed them to be tested for evidence of cancer. Then he'd start work on my tongue, cutting along the centre to get to the tumour and removing both the cancer itself and a cuff of healthy tissue around it by way of a safety zone. There were, he said, some imponderables. For instance I would certainly wake up with some sort of breathing tube poking down my nose into my windpipe and a feeding tube poking down my nose into my stomach, but depending on the amount of damage they did to my throat I might also have a tracheostomy – a plastic pipe pushed through a hole made in my neck and into my windpipe so that I could breathe – and a second pipe inserted directly through my abdomen and into my stomach through which I could be fed.

Suddenly the single operation to cut out the cancer had become five operations – the cancer removal, two neck dissections, a tracheostomy and a gastrectomy.

But there was more. Rhŷs Evans wasn't sure how much of my tongue he'd have to remove. If it was just so much and in just such a place he could simply sew up the hole; if it was so much and in a different place, well, it would be a job for the plastic surgeon, Nicholas Breach, who would be there helping at the operation anyway. Given the word, Breach would cut a wedge of my forearm out and sew it into the gap where part of my tongue had been removed. He'd then take some skin from my thigh to cover the hole in my forearm.

Seven ops in one. Whoopee.

I was scared again. Well of course I was: with the prospect of so much carnage being wreaked on so much of your body so would you have been. But I'd got used to not being properly scared; I'd become comfortable with my phoney stoicism. The problem was that with the camera running it seemed inappropriate to ask the scaredy-cat questions I really wanted to ask: have you done this before? When did you last lose a patient doing it? What are the chances of me needing all the optional extras? Will I live? Instead I asked stoical, practical questions: with a lump missing from my tongue would I be able to talk again, to broadcast, to sing? How long would recovery take? What were the chances of finding a tongue so rotten with cancer that the whole thing had to come out?

Rhŷs Evans' answers were, as is his way, optimistic ones. In my head, though, I heard: you will lose your tongue, you will never talk, you will recover after a long and painful convalescence and then, guess what? You'll die, because the whole thing was a waste of time.

I asked him what my chances were now that they so obviously weren't 92 per cent. This is the point, I know, at which professional statisticians will start grumbling. Yes, I understand that the original 92 per cent was still an accurate figure: the number of men who turn up at surgeries with my vague symptoms and live for five years afterwards is 92 in 100. But I was now a member of a different constituency: men of 44 with tongue cancer and local secondaries. It seemed reasonable to ask for some new statistics.

After rather less dissembling than I'd expected he settled on around 66 per cent or so – a two in three chance of being cured. It was meant to be reassuring, but for historical reasons I knew it couldn't possibly reassure.

Three and some years earlier we'd turned up to the hospital for the ultrasound test on the foetus who would become Cosima. The technician had a Wendyhouse approach to her job, and as she moved the probe around Nigella's distended stomach she'd look at the monitor and say 'Oooh! There's its little legs, and look! There's its little hands, and there's its little heart going pitter-patter...' and at the end of this we said so everything's OK then, right? And she said well actually no: there seem to be some little cysts on its little brain which are sometimes the precursor of a nasty chromosomal abnormality which has the baby dying of asphyxiation as it's being born.

In a state of shock we went up to the foetal medicine department where a doctor talked to us about a foetal blood test with a one in 100 chance of inducing a miscarriage balanced against the 1 in 250 chance that the cysts indicated something nasty.

As odds went they were reasonable ones and had I been standing in the bookie's thinking about putting money on a healthy baby there would have been no problem. But under the circumstances the odds were meaningless. In these situations all odds are the same odds, or rather evens. Either the worst will happen or it won't: the baby will die or it won't. The odds always feel like 50:50.

And as it was then so it was for me now. Either they'd cure me or they wouldn't. Everything was 50:50. When the official odds were 92 per cent they were really 50:50, and if the operation didn't work and the official odds dropped to 20 per cent or 10 per cent or worse, they'd still be 50:50.

The next day, *sans* cameras, we went for our last visit before the operation. Mr Breach, the consultant plastic surgeon, and, of course, the pre-eminent man in his etc. etc. etc., is a tall and rather old-fashioned sort of surgeon – rather like the pinstriped and jocular card from *Doctor in the House*. He keeps rooms in Portland Place, just along from the BBC and a few hundred yards away from the main medical drag in Harley Street, and wanted to see me for – well, I'm not quite sure what for. At the time I imagined that this was just one of the things that happened before big operations: you had a pleasant chat with the people who were going to be up to their elbows in your gore the next day.

If the Harley Street rooms were free of medical associations, Breach's Portland Place office was free of any associations at all. The featureless room could have been that of any professional, the entirely clear desk waiting for an accountant or a quantity surveyor to pop in with a calculator or a pile of bricks.

Breach went over the procedure again. From somewhere he found a piece of paper and a pen and started drawing diagrams of a face. As we knew, once the lower jaw had been split in two...

Hold on. What lower jaw split in two? We knew nothing about this.

Oh. He thought Mr Rhŷs Evans had explained. The easiest way

of getting to the very base of the tongue, given that no surgeon can get the whole of his scalpel-clutching fist into a patient's throat, is to saw along the bottom jaw from the point of the chin to just in front of the throat, prise the two halves apart and then work on the exposed tongue that way. He smiled and held his hands up in front of his face.

'It's just like opening a book.'

He mimed pulling the covers of a book apart and beamed again as if this analogy made it acceptable. It was quite a normal procedure, really. It would sew up neatly because he would cut the chin...

So far the news of the operation had been a smooth progression from the fact of its necessity through to the finer points of its procedure. It was frightening, sure, but it was somehow something I could understand, something I could imagine happening to me. As I'd understood it until now it was merely a question of cutting a nasty piece of me out and throwing it away. This, though, was something different. This was nightmare, bad horror movie, joke.

Was Breach sure this was the way Rhŷs Evans was going in? No: not absolutely certain, but it was the most likely way. As he was saying, the main incision would be...

Just a moment. There were questions I needed to ask. Would I?... was he?... did he think?... Damn! I couldn't think of a reasonable question. And then one mad one came to me. I have a cleft chin. It is the only part of me of which I've ever been proud. I may be overweight, and have short legs, and less hair than I once did, but Kirk Douglas and I have cleft chins. As far as I could tell, somebody was about to cut straight through the cleft. Would I still have my cleft chin at the end of the exercise?

In the scheme of things, and especially the disarrayed scheme in which I currently found myself, the future of my chin was of the smallest consequence. And yet here I was pleading for it to be saved.

Oddly, Breach seemed to understand. Or at least he didn't actually laugh out loud at my wretched vanity. I imagine plastic surgeons are used to such vanities. Never mind how he would split my lower jaw in two and pin it back together with lumps of titanium: this was how he'd make the cut which would hide the scar around my chin. He made a little zigzag shape on the diagram of the face. This was what his knife would do to my chin in 36 hours' time.

The next day I packed a grip with a pair of pyjamas, a wash-bag, an Apple Powerbook and the Alan Coren omnibus edition and Nigella and I drove to Fulham. I was booked in a day early to give them time to run the standard tests of my blood and my heart and my general condition, all of which felt pretty low. In Weston Ward in the newest of the hospital's blocks I had private room F – a Trusthouse Forte roadhouse of a room, with its almost bright walls and its framed art poster advertising some art poster artist's exhibition. High up on the wall was a small TV set and below it a wood-effect wardrobe. Sliding doors opened on to a balcony which ran along the whole of one side of the ward, along which promenaded pyjama'd men and women slowly pushing drip stands, talking to family and visitors, seemingly unaware – this being the head and neck ward – of their missing ears or cheeks or eyes or noses. Some had cream-coloured plastic tubes jutting forward from their throats: the tracheostomy I'd been promised.

The room had two beds: a narrow but fully adjustable hospital bed for me, and an even narrower put-u-up for Nigella, one of the bonuses of a private room being that she was allowed to stay

C

with me. My bed was surrounded by pipes and vacuum jars and emergency buttons. It was a bed for an ill person, a person who'd lost control of his own destiny and was in thrall to the doctors and nurses who knew how to suck the fluids into the vacuum jars and deliver the emergency oxygen and do whatever it was I wouldn't be able to do for myself after the operation.

There seemed no particular reason to get into my pyjamas, and so we lay on the bed watching television while a procession of nurses and technicians came and took samples of my blood and measured its pressure and did all those other little tasks which made me feel like a condemned man being made healthy for the gibbet.

Mr Patel, a handsome and rather shy young Indian registrar, came in and took us through the operation again. This time we got the six hours described in precise detail. Patel explained under precisely what circumstances they would or wouldn't open my jaw like a book, give me a tracheostomy, do any of the work which, in my mind at least, counted as a worst-case scenario.

'I think it's better if you understand what's happening before you start,' he said. 'It's easier to go through something when you know what it is you're going through.'

He was right: as Patel described the operation it became a matter of mechanics and hydraulics, of car maintenance rather than life saving. It's funny, though, how fashions change. It's not so long ago that most hospital doctors would have said that the best way to calm an anxious patient was to tell them as little as possible. Somebody told that their jaw will be prised open like a book can only worry; somebody told merely that a lump will be removed will go into the theatre in a state of tranquillity.

Until, of course, they wake up and feel the metal pins holding their jaw together and find they can't open their mouth to scream.

Either way, though, the fact is that it's impossible for the intact body to conceive of this sort of operation as anything but a mime. Like a child imagining death as eternity spent conscious in a wooden box, I could only think of the operation in its most mechanical terms.

At some point Mr Rhŷs Evans came to visit and I said that he hadn't actually mentioned the trick with the split jaw when we last spoke, and he said really? he was sure he had, although the cameras being on him as he described the operation hadn't helped. In any case, he said, he didn't know yet whether that was the way he'd go in. Somehow he managed to make me feel good about all the things that nobody yet knew – the way the surgery would be carried out, the number and nature of the tubes I'd have in me afterwards, the chances I had of living through all of this.

I asked whether I was needed for anything else that day and Rhŷs Evans looked around the medical team which had come with him into the room, and they all said that no, they'd taken all the bits of me they needed to take for the time being. We'd already agreed that once the fluid samples had been taken and the tests run, I could go off until bedtime, but I asked whether there was any real reason why I had to be back that night given that I wasn't needed to play my part in the drama until midday tomorrow. Knowing about hospital bureaucracy I already knew the answer, but again Rhŷs Evans looked around. Was there any particular reason why I had to be back until the next morning? Nobody could think of one. To my amazement I was let out. As long as I was back by 8 a.m. I had a temporary reprieve.

Nigella and I went home and decided to book a table

somewhere congenial for what would, in any circumstance, be our last proper dinner for a while. Ruthie Rogers, a good friend and so often a solace in so many ways, gave us a table at her River Cafe, and we ate well, and laughed, and drank just enough, and afterwards we walked along the Thames in the dark, arm in arm. We came to a brightly lit school hall of some sort where, on the other side of the glass, a couple of dozen men and women of every age were involved in some sort of ballroom dancing lesson. I can't tell you why we both found watching these happy people bumping into each other so incredibly moving, but we stood by the river and smiled at each other.

We walked back chattering about everything except the operation. It wasn't a question of repressing, or blocking or avoiding, just that with so little time left for us to be normal together, we wanted to make the most of it.

We drove home and lay together in our bed for what was to be the last time as the couple we had been for eight years.

Tomorrow I would become somebody else.

Chapter 8

C

I had fallen among nurses.

There are various versions of what happened when I came round. Nigella's is that she turned up and found me dozing, clutching a clipboard on which were scrawled the words 'Absolutely fucking wonderful. And you?', which heavy irony was apparently aimed at some poor nurse who'd seen I'd come to and asked how I was feeling.

Bywater's slightly more surreal version is that he found a scribbled note which he swears preceded any other and which read, simply, 'Nebbish', the Yiddish word to describe a person to whom wretched things are always happening. I like Bywater's version better, describing, as it does, a man who rises to the majesty of Yiddish *in* post-operative *extremis*, but given that Nigella arrived so soon after I came round in what I still think of as Intensive Care but which hospitals, just to rub it in, now call the High Dependency Unit, she probably has it right.

In fact I had slept through the night and woke for the first time at five the next morning, and my true first scribble said 'Where's Nigella'. Nigella had been sent home the night before on the basis that she had some rough nights in front of her and could probably use all the sleep she could get.

Certainly when she turned up I remember writing a second note which read – 'chillingly', Nigella now says – 'Can you see a tongue in there'. She looked, and then passed me her powder-compact mirror so that I could look myself.

There was a tongue. There was more than a tongue. As a nine-month-pregnant mother is with child, so my mouth was with tongue. It was filled with livid pink tongue from roof to floor and covering the teeth from side to side. Bloated tongue was all there was.

C

I looked more carefully, bringing the mirror towards my face because I couldn't move the tongue any further forward. Or backward. Big as my tongue was, it was completely immobile. It was also, I noticed, slightly more swollen on one side than the other, and along a diagonal line from front right to back left there was a valley which dipped down to the invisible sutures where the two halves had been sewn back together. It was also pointed at the front, like the tongue of some unknown reptile.

Thinking back I realised there would have to be a tongue in there: the last thing I did before we left for home the day before was sign the standard form consenting to the operation on which I'd scribbled a rider specifying that they'd have to wake me up if it became apparent that a total glossectomy – a full removal of the tongue – was needed. Rhŷs Evans had considered it entirely unlikely: it would only be necessary if the cancer had spread to the jaw and gums and, as importantly, to the veins and arteries which would communicate it to other, more distant, parts of the body. My feeling was that if things had gone that far then for the first time in all of this I might have a choice – between living for n months or years with a tongue or living for slightly longer without one. It might well have been that I'd have gone for a short life but a gabby one.

But if a tongue was there – or part of one, at least – what was missing?

I looked down at my forearm. It was complete. Both of them were. No plastic surgery. Which might mean – I held up the mirror again: my chin was swollen almost beyond recognition, but it was whole, and at the tip of it was the distended remembrance of a cleft. Small mercies indeed, but I'd stopped being surprised by the events I now found merciful. So far I knew this: I'd had enough tongue removed to cause the remnant to swell up like a toy balloon, but not so much had been taken that I needed plastic surgery. They'd gone in through my mouth rather than through my chin and – and I was alive.

All of which probably makes me sound rather more alive than I felt.

I remember that one of my last thoughts had been that all else aside, the thing which would scare me most on waking was being too dazed to know why I was dazed, why I was in pain, why I was in this strange bed connected by tubes to God knows what equipment. In fact I realised where I was and why as quickly as one does on waking in a strange hotel room after a night on the booze. It seemed reasonable, for instance, that I had to write a note to the nurse rather than talk to her. As for the pain, well there was none to speak of. There was discomfort, certainly, because like some groggy Gulliver I was pinioned to the bed by a dozen tubes, but no pain. At the time I think I believed this was a matter of luck rather than the morphine that one of the tubes was, I later learned, pumping into me.

The tubes were all over me. Two were poked into holes in either side of my neck, draining fluid away from where the lymph glands had been removed; one entered my windpipe via my nostril so that I could get some air past the tongue which was filling the whole of my oral cavity; one entered my stomach via my other nostril and would eventually be connected to the bottles from which dripped my foul liquid meals. There was a tube sending antibiotics into my arm and another one sending glucose into the other arm and a third feeding an arm with morphine. There was also a tube connected to a catheter shoved up my urethra and carrying away my urine. (Here's a tip for the gents in the audience. If anyone ever asks if he can poke a catheter up your urethra and leave it there for a few days, tell him no. They will say it doesn't hurt and express surprise when, on pulling it out a few days later, they have to scrape you off the ceiling. Avoid.) Finally I had a line connected at one end to a plastic ring around my finger and at the other to the familiar beeping machine which monitored various cardiovascular attributes.

There were other tubes draped around me waiting for their turn: oxygen lines, suction tubes, tracheostomy tube.

And this was what life was like after the low-key, no plastic surgery version of the operation. I couldn't imagine what it would be like if on top of the partial glossectomy I was also dealing with a forearm transplant. (Some months later Bywater, who'd been so gung-ho about the usefulness of every promised aspect of the operation, told me that this was a good one to avoid and let slip that he knew somebody who'd been split up the chin and that he was in desperately serious pain for a couple of weeks afterwards.) In fact I learned subsequently that the choice was wider than that between split-chin and down-the-throat. Depending on my surgeon, on his skill, and on what he found when he opened my mouth up, there were any number of ways of getting to the tumour. They could have made a hole in the side of my face and gone in that way, or come from just above my throat and through the bottom of my jaw. Both those methods would have involved dealing harshly with a major lingual nerve and effectively paralysing one side of the remainder of my tongue for good. As it was, I'd lost a large lump of tongue, but the rest of it still had its full complement of nerves.

I woke, I dozed off, I woke, I dozed off.

Although I had been booked to go into surgery at midday, I finished up being trollied into the lift down to the basement operating theatre an hour or so late: Rhŷs Evans had a couple of quick procedures to knock off before mine and one of them took slightly longer than expected. By this time, though, I was pre-med-ed up to my eyeballs and didn't much mind either way.

The BBC had got permission from the hospital for its cameras to follow me from my room to the door of the ante-room to the theatre where I'd be given the anaesthetic. For all the right televisual reasons Olivia Lichtenstein had filled rather too many of my last pre-operative minutes with penetrating 'How do you feel' questions, and actually arriving at the theatre had been something of a relief. But then the whole affair felt like a scene from a TV play: with my head pinioned on to the trolley I would only see people – anaesthetists, nurses, wives – when they poked their heads into my field of vision. In the last moments before the anaesthetist got to me I was more concerned with the camera shot than I was with what was about to happen to me.

Until now all my medical dealings had been with doctors. Now I was bed-bound I saw my doctors only when they did their morning and evening rounds but the nurses were around all the time. On the High Dependency Unit I had a side ward – mainly in deference to the cameras, lest they catch a glimpse of another patient – and a collection of smiling uniformed men and women who slipped in and out to change drips, note the readings of the various bits of machinery and generally make sure I was still alive. A day after I came round I was given my slippers and dressing gown and sent for a walk around the main ward supported between Nigella and one of the nurses on the basis that the less time I was highly dependent the better.

The nurse suggested I walk to the end of the corridor and back. Instead I shuffled to the end of the corridor, past the hospital's hairdressing salon, across the landing above the gloomy

C

painting of sometime benefactor Mrs Burdett-Coutts and the leather sofa on which I'd occasionally see crying families just given the worst news, past the entrance of my home ward, and back to the unit again. This was generally judged by the nurses to be the long-distance walk of a superman, of a man so nearly recovered from the major surgery of a few hours ago as to be miraculous. I was sure they said that to all the tubed-up boys just out of theatre, but I felt immensely proud of myself.

My trip round the rest of the ward gave the me the first real sign of what the deal was here. It was the quietest hospital ward I'd ever seen either as patient or visitor. In a permanent twilight everyone was either recovering from recent surgery or in some relapsing state which called for intensive care. In one bed was an Arab woman, rendered un-Semitically whey-faced, and unconscious for all the time I was on the ward, obviously sinking fast and surrounded by female relatives moaning slightly; across from her was a man, alone and unvisited, recovering silently from some major piece of surgery which had left him as heavily tubed and bandaged as me. Patients would be slipped in and out of the ward under cover of dark, but all of them *looked* like patients: bandaged and be-tubed, yes, but also with faces drawn, staring eyes lacklustre, cheeks sunken. These were people in real trouble, and for the first time I felt as if I were in trouble too.

On the second day Mr Rhŷs Evans appeared, surrounded by his corps of registrars and housemen and women, to give me details of how much trouble I was in.

It could have been worse.

The tumour and the surrounding tissue turned out to be the size of a golfball, which meant we'd moved on to a whole new lump metaphor scale. When they took the lump out of my neck and still thought it was benign, they told me it was the size of a clementine. But now my lumps were malignant we'd moved away from the fruit lump scale – grape, kumquat, clementine, melon – and over to the more worrying sporting lump scale on which men were felled by lumps the size of rugby balls. How everyone could have missed an extraneous lump that big was beyond me, but this wasn't a time to start complaining. Even, of course, if I'd been in any position to complain.

The good news was found in my lymph glands. As each gland was popped out of my neck during the operation, it was rushed down to Dr Cyril Fisher (a man I'd not yet met but who was to become one of my favourite Marsdenites) in the histopathology department. Fisher and his team would immediately freeze the gland, slice off some microscopically thin slivers in a microtome, douse each sliver in a stain which would show its constituent parts more readily, shove it under a microscope, determine whether it was cancerous or not and send the glad word back up to the theatre.

All the glands on the left side of my neck – which is to say the ones which had been irradiated over the previous six weeks – were entirely cancer free. There were a couple which had a few cancerous cells on the right-hand side, but there was a buffer zone of cancer-free glands at the top and bottom of the chain of glands. This meant that although the cancer had spread locally it hadn't spread to any distant sites. Or, at least, if it had it wasn't via the usual lymphatic route.

Not all the news was good, though. Rhŷs Evans and his team hadn't been able to take out as much of a cuff of healthy tissue around the tumour as they had wished. He spoke equivocally, and I couldn't quite be sure whether I was right in my suspicion that this meant there was an area where there was no cuff at all. This would be doubly worrying: worrying on the first count

C

because everything at the moment was worrying, and on the second because leaving a big margin is the only way a surgeon can be fairly certain of having excised the whole of a tumour.

Either way this meant that once I was sufficiently recovered from my operation I had to have a second six-weeks' worth of radiotherapy, this time to the right-hand side of my neck and to most of my tongue, in order to mop up any stray cancer cells which the knife might have missed.

I groaned. Those last days of the first radiotherapy sessions were still close enough for me to be able to smell the depression and the frustration. I wasn't sure that I could face another lot.

Like there was a choice.

On the third day they told me again about the body's miraculous recuperative powers and talked about moving me back to Weston Ward. Bywater popped in on the way to the Chelsea arts club and looked at the dials on the bits of machinery.

'Olympian,' he said, as if sarcastically. 'Look at that heart rate. Look at that blood pressure.'

I beamed to myself. I knew it was Bywater's magnificent overstatement – he has a way of conferring compliments by offering them as insults – but the truth was that with my lungs cleared of Marlborough fumes and my frame free of a few stone I was probably in a better condition to undergo eight hours of surgery than I had been for years. My heart was strolling at a reasonable 60-odd beats a minute, my blood was calm in my slack veins. Sick as I was, I was also, and possibly for the first time in my life, healthy.

I beamed because that was the only immediate way I could communicate, and even then the bruising in my mouth meant it was a fairly crooked beam. The most immediate cause of my dumbness was the tube passing down my windpipe and stopping my vocal cords from moving. Until the tube was removed I'd have no idea of how impaired my speech would be. Certainly the pre-operative impression given by Rhŷs Evans and Breach was that I'd have, as it were, the conversational equivalent of a slight limp for a while. A few days before the operation I'd had a call from Stephanie Kingham, a speech therapist who had worked at the Marsden and was now in private practice. She'd been reading the column and listening to me on radio and said that she'd known that there was some problem with my tongue: to her professional ear it had sounded 'tethered'.

We'd talked about what sort of therapy I'd need and how impaired my speech was likely to be, and although the degree of impairment would obviously be dependent on the amount of tongue they took out and the route they used to get at it, she seemed to think there was no reason why I shouldn't be broadcasting again three months later in November, when I was booked to present the last series of *Fourth Column* and another series of *The People's Parliament* on Channel 4. And now even though I couldn't utter a word, the fact that there had been no need for plastic surgery suggested that this would, indeed, be a temporary state of affairs.

I was wrong – again – as it happened, but meanwhile I had a clipboard and pen. A couple of days later I had something better than that: Douglas Adams had used his status as Britain's Greatest Comic Science Fiction Writer to borrow an Apple Powerbook for me from the makers, which allowed me to play Stephen Hawking by typing my irritable thoughts on to the screen and having them read out in a robotic voice on the computer's speaker. It seems to work for Hawking, but

C

whenever I typed anything the person to whom I was cyber-talking would always wander over and watch the screen and read... the... words... out... loud... in... a... bright... and... infuriating... monotone... as... I... typed... them.

On the fourth day I returned to Room F at the Weston Ward. They came and told me in the morning that I'd be going back, and so Nigella and I collected up my things, hooked up the tubed accessories to a mobile hatstand-on-wheels affair, and started to walk the few yards down the corridor to the ward. It wasn't until some days later that I learned that I was the first person in recent memory to walk out of the High Dependency Unit and that everyone else left in a wheelchair. Or, of course, in a box.

The news should have made me cheerful, but my mood had swung and all I could think of was the irony. It's taken me all these years to discover that I have the constitution of an ox, and here I am maybe about to die.

But mood swings go both ways. I had my own bed in my own room; it was summer and the sun was shining; every afternoon there was *Columbo* on the TV suspended above the bed, every night and morning there was Nigella looking beautiful and breathing gently in the put-u-up on the other side of the small room. If God wasn't exactly in his heaven then He had surely popped out for only a short while.

In my hypochondriacal days, just a lifetime or so ago at the start of the year, the prospect of a bed in hospital seemed to me to be an ideal one. I remember there used to be a sitcom on the box called *Only When I Laugh* which had as its premise the idea that a pair of malingerers had conspired to stay in adjoining hospital beds for long enough to construct a couple of seasons of sitcoms

around them. There seemed to be nothing odd about an illness –
who can remember what it was or whether it was ever specified?
– chronic enough to keep them in hospital but benign enough to
allow them to take an active part in each week's plot. More, there
seemed nothing odd about them *wanting* to stay in hospital for
as long as possible, in a bed made up for them daily, with piles
of books at one side, a TV at eye level, friendly nurses on call 24
hours a day.

And from my hypochondriacal point of view there was the
added advantage of having qualified medical people right on
hand to thump my chest, or inject the adrenalin, or explain that
the pain was only indigestion.

But that wasn't how it felt now. Rather than comforted, I felt
dislocated. This was the time I wanted to be at home, in our bed,
with the kids in the next room. This bed was uncomfortable with
its slippery plastic mattress cover below the sheets and the
pillows which wouldn't settle properly.

And then there was the food. I wouldn't be able to eat in the
normal way, I knew, for some weeks although I wasn't quite sure
at the time what form my not being able to eat would eventually
take. Instead the feeding tube which entered my stomach
through my nostril was hooked up to something called *Jevity* – a
name coined by somebody with a shaky grasp on etymology and
who thought 'longevity' had its true root at the arse-end of the
word. Jevity comes in half-litre bottles, is beige in the way that
old ladies' knickers in Fenwick's are beige, and is 500
malodorous calories' worth of assorted fats, fibres, proteins,
triglycerides, vitamins and other life-sustaining oddments. The
half-litre took two hours to be pumped into me by a little blue
electric pump that was forever tripping over its own whirring
innards and becoming blocked and sending out a shrill beep to

C

alert the nurses and to wake me up. I needed 2,000 calories a day, or four bottles of Jevity, to give me the energy to get over the operation; it meant some eight hours a day hooked up to the pump. One day, I was told brightly by a nurse, my stomach would be strong enough to receive Jevity pumped in at twice the speed. It seemed a pretty miserable goal to aim for.

And so I spent the days in a state of enforced surliness with the pump whirring food down my nose, the tubes draining off all my excess fluids and keeping the morphine topped up. Jemima would come in with a tiny video camera and take footage of me looking irritable, Bywater would come in and tell me about his love life, Ruthie came in a couple of times with some videos and a pair of beautiful blue crumpled linen trousers. I tapped out a couple of snarling columns on the lap-top complaining about my situation and readers started sending me *nil desperandum* letters care of the hospital. I scribbled messages to everyone who'd read them complaining about everything: the painkillers not turning up on time, the painkillers turning up too early, the suction tube not working properly... and what I was really complaining about was being in hospital.

The problem with major surgery – any surgery – is that there is no real way of anyone telling you how it will be when you come round. I'd had conversations with various of the medical people and although nobody goes into any great detail about the tubes and the bed, I had some idea of the wreckage that my physical form would suffer – that I'd be cut, and bandaged, and scarred. And I'd guessed that I'd feel pretty miserable, although misery wasn't really the term to describe the mixture of drug-dampened pain, irritation and physical constraint. But nobody can tell you how it feels to be that post-operative person, the person who is lying there waiting for the new chapter to start and with no idea of how that chapter will read. I knew that everything that had been done to me would have a permanent effect, but I couldn't say what that effect – on my constitution, my looks, my voice, my career, my persona – would be. I lay there and contemplated the new me and was frustrated by the shallowness of contemplation which was possible.

By the third day back on the ward my tubage had lessened somewhat. They'd taken the drains out of my swollen neck and now I could walk to the lavatory I didn't need the catheter. The regular morphine had been replaced by an occasional fix, but most of the pain relief came from an assortment of lesser analgesics. Above all, the breathing tube which had been flattening my vocal tubes was taken out and I could talk.

'Talk', I say. I could honk is what I could do. I could splutter. I could dribble. Occasionally I could get somebody to understand a word. But with much of the back of my tongue missing and the rest of it swollen where the Y-shaped slash had been stitched together, I couldn't talk. Each morning I would make up a solution of disinfectant mouthwash and scrub around my mouth with a piece of foam on a stick, using my fingers to lift my flaccid and unmuscled tongue out of the way to get at the floor of my mouth.

Again, I might have guessed that the immediate effect of the operation would have been that my speech would be impaired; the other side-effects were entirely unguessable. I hadn't considered, for instance, saliva. Although I should by now have been short at least one saliva gland following the radiotherapy, the others were making up for the loss and I was producing litres of the stuff. Pre-operatively that would have been no problem: we swallow the saliva that is extraneous to that which we need for eating and general lubrication. But before we can swallow we have to get the liquid to the back of the throat, a fairly basic glottal manoeuvre undertaken by the muscly tongue. Not mine, though. I had no way of getting the saliva to my throat. It would gather in pools at the front of my mouth and at the sides and leak out when I opened my mouth. Worse, it wasn't the thin liquid that constitutes most of the world's saliva deposits, but, thanks to the radiotherapy and the operation, a thick and glutinous jelly. I would have washed out my mouth with cold water, if I'd been able to swallow and if I'd been allowed water to drink. The only way of getting rid of it was to stick the suction tube at the side of my bed into the maw and poke around until it was all cleaned out and the jar of evil-looking gloop into which the tube ran was a little fuller.

All of which might have been a little easier if I could have slept, for when I thought of hospital beds it was sleeping that I really imagined: life as a single extended lie-in with nobody to kick you in the shins and ask you to make a cup of tea. But every time I got near sleep my bloated tongue would loll back into my throat and I'd come back to woozy wakefulness, gagging. Despite the sleeping pills and the morphine I didn't get more than an hour's sleep for most of the time I was in hospital.

That time had started off as 'Ten days to two weeks' in Rhŷs Evans' estimation, and then fixed itself at two weeks in his conversation as if the ten-day option had never been there, and on the day before I went under he mentioned in passing that, of course, after two or three weeks in hospital... The way things were going it was a matter of time before they were talking in months.

By the fifth day – the second on Weston Ward after three on the High Dependency Unit – I couldn't face the thought of the nine days – at least – which were to come. I was going stir crazy. I wasn't sleeping, couldn't talk, couldn't think. I would lie there watching 3 a.m. turn into 4 and into 5 and then 6, listening to the small night-time noises of the ward outside, of the Fulham Road and the dawn-waking pigeons, to the whirr of my feeding pump, and I would seethe. And as I seethed the plastic sheeting beneath me would crackle in the heat.

At five in the morning of that fifth day I lost it. I hadn't had any painkillers that night, not least because I was taking them on an as-needed basis and I hadn't remembered to ask for any. When the nurse popped her head round to check on me I exploded. Why had I not been given any painkillers? What was going on? Didn't they have any bloody pillows that didn't have that sweat-making plastic covering? The nurse got it full force and left to get me some pain relief. Nigella, lying on the floor like a stereotypical Indian wife, sprang up from the doze which was as much as she ever managed in hospital.

I screamed, literally, and started thumping the walls with my fist. I couldn't stay here any longer. I was going. Now.

In my mad rage I started getting dressed, pulling out tubes as I went. Nigella rushed to get a nurse and tell her that her husband, still hooked up to a few tubes, still eating and breathing post-operatively, was crashing around his room, trying to leave the hospital.

The nurse strode into my room. She was an older woman, unflappable, with the look of one who had seen more idiots try to discharge themselves than I'd had hot dinners. Not that I'd had many of those recently. Fine: if I wanted to discharge myself, that was up to me and, as I knew, there was nothing they could do about it. On the other hand, I could wait a couple of hours for the consultant to turn up on his early morning rounds, and talk with him about my problem.

C

Mad as I was I understood that it would be madder not to wait.

I lay on the bed watching the breakfast news and with my seethe burbling away in the background, while Nigella, still unsure whether this was a temporary rage or the start of some more permanent flippery, humoured me gently.

At 8 a.m. Mr Breach turned up: Rhŷs Evans was away that week and Breach was taking the ward rounds. I assumed that he'd been primed before he got to my room: certainly he approached me with the smiling equanimity of one who knows the conversation may go in any direction. More, with his team around him there was some hint that I was presenting a particular clinical problem – post-operative cancer patient goes berserk and starts beating walls – from which they could all learn.

We went through the usual morning routine: check swelling, look at vital signs, talk about pain control – and then Breach asked what the problem seemed to be in a way which implied the words 'old boy' at the end of the sentence without actually saying them. I told him. About the lack of sleep, and the crackling bed, and the feeling of dislocation. And then, because put like this my list of complaints seemed absurdly short for all the madness I was attaching to it, I told him again.

Breach shrugged and turned to the nurse in attendance. What exactly was the hospital doing for me that couldn't be done at home? I was breathing on my own and the two drains had been taken out of my neck a couple of days earlier. All my pain relief now came in tablet form and I was due to get my last antibiotic drip that afternoon. The only tube that had to stay in was the one running down my nostril and into my stomach carrying the Jevity. Would it be possible, Breach asked, for me to borrow a pump from the hospital and take it and a few dozen bottles of

Jevity and go home?

There was a very brief silence while everyone considered this as if it were some sort of physics problem which they knew they should be able to answer but still couldn't quite compute. The nurse gave the answer, and a very Marsden answer it was too in its patient-centredness: no – there was absolutely no reason at all why what was being done for me here couldn't be done at home provided the district nurse was given due warning.

That afternoon I went home, almost to die within the fortnight.

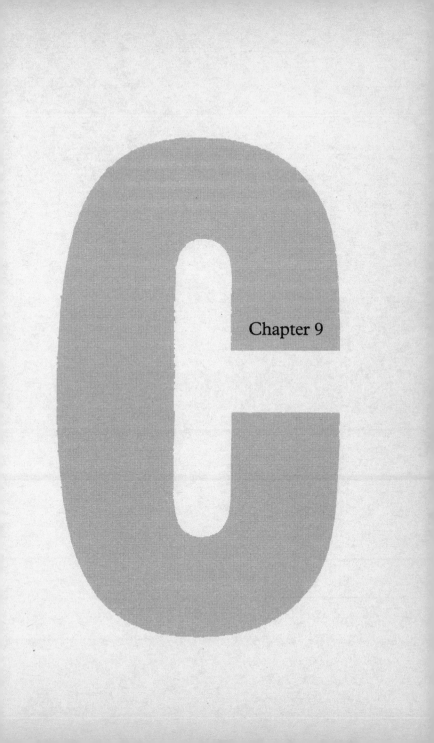

Chapter 9

J ust as there are those who still believe that notwithstanding the disappearance of the Berlin Wall, the flotation of the rouble and the departure of most of the staff of *Marxism Today* to the leader offices of the national broadsheet press, Marx was as right now as ever he was in 1848 or 1917 or 1968, so in our post-Freudian age Nigella is one of the last of the unreconstructed Freudians. I believe that Freud's heart was in the right place and that he cobbled together some reasonable theories out of some dodgy observations, which is more than can be said for Jung or Adler, but Nigella is a Freudian like the Pope is a Catholic. OK: bad analogy for it's not that she treats Freud as a religious figure but that within certain marginal aspects of the human condition – all human emotions and interaction, for instance – she believes that his theories explain most things.

Not long ago she offered me a personal Freudian theory which she assumed I wouldn't agree with. There was some level, she said, at which my partially missing tongue was the equivalent of my being castrated. Perhaps it wasn't an absolute equivalent, but I certainly saw her point.

As the swelling of the tongue started to go down it became apparent that this wasn't, after all, the glottal equivalent of a broken leg: it needed more than bed rest and my keeping my weight off it to get back to its old form. If, indeed, there was any chance of it getting back to its old form.

Those of us not employed in any of the anatomical professions think of the tongue as the flap which extends from the top of the throat to the front of the teeth or, if we stick the flap out, a little further still. But the great mass of the tongue is behind and beneath that flap, the muscular stanchion which roots it to the throat, and it was mainly from this that the tumorous golf ball had been snatched. The tongue is muscle: it is infinitely movable

C

along its length. To say 'tea' you need to be able to touch the tip of the tongue to the front of the roof of the mouth; to say 'cocoa' you need to be able to do the same at the back of the mouth. The sounds of the language require us to poke the tongue forwards, bend it in the middle, flick it up, use it to scrape the back of the teeth.

I could do none of these things. My tongue had been dragged back to cover the golf ball-sized hole and I couldn't get its tip to touch my teeth at the front. It wouldn't move up, or down or sideways; indeed the only voluntary movement I could see in the mirror was a slight twitch at the back of the tongue – perfect for the East London glottal stop which I'd spent a lifetime trying to get rid of, but pretty useless for much else.

To say I lived by my voice would be overstating the case, but not by much. Certainly in the most literal sense between a third and a half of my working week involved throwing my voice around one sort of broadcasting studio or another, and another third involved my phoning people up to ask them questions the answers to which I could quote in a paper or magazine. If nothing else, I understood that my living for the next few months would have to be made from writing about my own thoughts rather than asking others for theirs.

But it wasn't the professional problem which left me feeling impotent. We all have self-images which may be based on a fallacious reading of how we present ourselves to others but which are, nevertheless, the way we believe ourselves to be. Like a page 3 girl who believes that she is described entirely by her breasts so I believe my personality to be almost entirely manifest in what I say and the way that I say it, that people respond to me not because I am good or kind or have a face which encourages response, but because of the words I speak. There is part of me which believes, for instance, that I have never taken a woman to bed but that I talked her there, that I have never got a job but that I talked my way into it.

The fact is that I *am* talking: talking is what I do. Fair enough, I'm not Oscar Wilde or Moss Hart but to have a riposte or a description or a question sitting there on my lips waiting to be shot into the conversational mêlée and not being able to shoot it was emasculating. And though there may be plenty who say that my old verbal incontinence was a bad thing, that it made me facile and unthinking, I enjoyed being the person I was pre-operatively and I found now that there were times when not only did I not enjoy the condition I found myself in, but that I didn't enjoy being the person I now was. Pre-operatively I was profligate with words, throwing away jokes and cracks and little sarcasms to fill up the spaces between thoughts. Now no word was wasted. I used the words I needed to use but there was a second busy dialogue playing – but only to me – in the background.

I realised what was happening when one day Nigella said something with which I agreed and to which I meant to respond 'Absolutely!' But the word which came out was 'Yes'. It was a footling thing, I knew, but the John Diamond who says 'yes' is a different person from the one who says 'absolutely'.

Worse, I found myself having depressed and depressing thoughts about who this made me. I found myself forced to entertain the thought from time to time: would the people I love love me, know me, have taken trouble with me, if this is I how I was when they first met me? Would my friends, friends in whom I've never had a doubt, have become my friends if when we first met I'd been a wounded, honking mute unable to respond to the simplest question without dribbling? Would I be with Nigella,

C

come to that? Would I have the kids?

I knew I had entered the twitchy land of Jimmy Stewart in *It's a Wonderful Life*, but I also knew that the answer to most of those questions was almost certainly 'no'. It had to be: I didn't have any friends who were honking dribblers and I was the only honking dribbler among my friends' friends. Perhaps it should be otherwise: perhaps we should all have gone out and clutched the halt and the lame to our urbane bosoms and discovered that underneath the superficial fact of their deafness or dumbness they were born-again Woody Allens – but we didn't. And so, I deduced, it must follow that I was not now the person my friends befriended, my wife married.

It was, I understood, an equation born in late-night depression, for once one starts totting up the what-ifs in a middle-aged life one can get badly, if temporarily, hurt. But the fact remained: I was not me any more. That my friends seemed to be willing to do almost anything for me was, I believed in those mad moments, almost worse: they were responding to who I was before the operation rather than who I had become after it. I believed then that in a month or two the various therapies would be over and that I would be the chattering classes' Mr Facile all over again, but meanwhile this is what disease does to us. It wrecks our faces and our voices and any talents we may have lying around, and then it makes us separately depressed so that we're unable to deal with the wreckage.

And so, back in the comfort of my own home, I started moping. I was still in pain but without the hospital's timetabled regime I found that I was skipping painkillers because I couldn't remember when I'd taken the last lot. For much of the time I was still attached to the Jevity pump which I'd sped up slightly but which still took the best part of six hours of the day away from me.

I started behaving like a crotchety invalid – snapping at Nigella and the children, throwing the occasional wild-eyed wobbler. Nigella got the brunt of it and, worse, suffered uncomplainingly. She had been the one who had got up at 6 a.m. every morning we shared a room in hospital so that she would be at home when the children woke, but, hey, I was the one with cancer and never mind that the physical and mental toll it took on Nigella was vast: how could she complain?

I would go into long rages: I'd imagine myself suddenly able to drink a cup of coffee or eat a soft cheese sandwich and when I found I couldn't – why did I think I could? – hurling the coffee or the sandwich across the room. The Gestalt merchants would have said this was just the sort of anger therapy I needed, but it was lousy therapy for Nigella and the children.

Worse, though, was the depression. Every apparent step forward, every signpost on the way to possible recovery seemed to induce in me a massive despondency. The ending of the first radiotherapy sessions had; so had the operation which was due to cut out my cancer. I wouldn't see anybody either personally or – as in the phrase so beloved of doctors 'It might help if you *saw* somebody?' – professionally, thus making sure that Nigella continued to get the brunt of my misery. A week or so after I got back I unilaterally declined any further treatment at all: I didn't care what effect it had on my illness, I said, I just couldn't bear the state I was in.

And I couldn't. Somehow it seemed worse at home. In hospital being disabled seemed a reasonable state of affairs: at home it turned me into a disabled person, unable to eat or drink or speak properly.

And even worse still: I was clinging to my illness. Apart from

C

Nigella and the children, it was the only constant, the only thing I really understood. My writing about it changed: I was writing to protect something of which I was jealous, something which was starting to describe me in the way that my speaking had described me in the old days.

My relationship with my cancer had changed for another reason too.

When I first started writing about the illness I was, as far as I'd known, a voice alone. I'd never denied that I was writing for entirely selfish reasons and that the writing had been the perfect therapy. I had known, although not well, Martyn Harris who had written in the *Telegraph* about his own terminal cancer a couple of years earlier and thus I knew enough to counter those readers who wrote to tell me that I was the first to break the taboo. But suddenly cancer seemed to be everywhere. *The Sunday Times* devoted a whole issue of its colour magazine to it; Michael Korda's tale of his prostate cancer, *Man to Man*, was all over the place, and, most difficultly, Ruth Picardie was writing about her cancer in the *Observer* magazine.

I say most difficultly because Ruth, the mother of two-year-old twins, was dying of her illness. It made me feel a fraud. Here was I swinging between jokiness and self-pity each week over a cancer which only had a small chance of carrying me off, and here was a real sufferer who could write about her chemotherapy, her grieving family, her imminent death with a good humour which I felt, in my current bad humour, made my own jocularity look forced.

What is most telling of my feelings at the time is not that I felt fraudulent but that I saw Ruth as a rival in some mad way. I was the journalist with cancer, for God's sake, and here she was, waltzing on to the page with her own terminal disease and showing me up. Worse: here she was *making me cry*. I confessed this to a couple of friends who were mutual to Ruth and myself and they told me I was mad, which is comforting in hindsight even if it wasn't at the time.

But still I had the feeling that I had become part of some sort of bandwagon. Not long after Ruth started writing her epistles from her deathbed I received an e-mail from Roy Greenslade, a close friend who had been my editor years ago when I was on the *Mirror* and who was now the most astute of the newspaper media commentators. He was writing a piece for the *Guardian* on Ruth and me: could I answer some questions? The piece appeared the next week as a summation of all the praise the readers had been writing to me for months now. I found it impossible to deal with, not least because I didn't feel like the person Greenslade was writing about.

The children seemed to take it all in relatively good part. It was easy enough for Bruno: at just over a year old if he knew what I was saying it had nothing to do with whether I said it in purest BBC or in my current voice. For Cosima, at getting on for four, it was rather different. She'd been in to see me in hospital a couple of times and had been generally fêted by the nurses and although she realised I was in some discomfort she had no actual reason to believe that there was any danger involved. Come to that, she wasn't really capable of understanding what those dangers might really mean even if we'd thought it proper to explain them to her. She understood that I'd hurt my neck and that this had affected my speech. And in fact she had no problem with not being able to understand me as well as she once had: when she missed a word she simply said 'what?' even if the word she missed was in the middle of some telling off or another.

C

But occasionally my illness seemed to inform some nascent hypochondria she was developing. She would announce, with no apparent reason, that she had a bad throat, or a sore neck, or that her doll did. It was understandable enough: not so long ago she'd been the centre of attention at home, but first came her brother to share that attention and then for some reason which had something to do with his throat, her father was getting all the notice.

I was still sleeping badly. I'd doze and then just as the doze would be transformed into proper sleep, I'd come round with a jolt. What was happening, it seemed, was that in that transformation my already post-operatively slack muscles would slacken even further: my tongue would loll back, my epiglottis close off, and I would be conscious of not taking in as much air. Part of the problem was, according to Rhŷs Evans, that like a fifth of the population I had a so-called 'infantile' epiglottis: a tightly bunched little thing which choked off part of the airway at the best of times. The nights became a tedious round of dozing and waking, never sleeping. But at least I was dozing and waking in my own bed, with Nigella next to me.

And then a week or so after I came home I woke from not quite sleeping at 2 a.m., unable to breathe. That was OK: I'd woken like this before. Normally a cough would clear the gunge from around my tongue, break the seal, and I'd breathe again. Not this time though. I coughed and coughed, and weak little coughs they were with my lungs blocked off. And so I screamed to Nigella.

'I can't breathe.'

I'd like to be able to tell you that in my moment of need my crippled tongue came good. It didn't. What I screamed out was

'Ny Naunt Reive.'

Nigella leapt out of bed not knowing what to do. I was squatting on the floor at the end of the bed, one hand beating the wall, the other clutched to my throat. She offered a glass of water, a steadying hand.

'Het a Hnblnse!' I screamed. And again. This time Nigella understood; she rang for an ambulance.

'I'm dying,' I said, which, oddly, was an arrangement of sounds my mouth could deal with. It came out as 'I'm dying.'

I certainly believed I was dying and up to a point I was. Until now, close though my encounters with death had been in my own mind, they had something of an abstract quality. Having cancer and its accompanying statistical chance of death isn't the same as being on one's deathbed. Over these past months I had been conscious some of the time that I might die soon, and there are chapters of what you've read so far where I could accurately convey my state of mind only by adding the words 'and the thing is, I might die!' to the end of every sentence and having it printed in a 16-point Hysterical typeface. But for most of the time I felt as conscious as I was before the diagnosis of being on a track which would end at a terminus. The track just felt shorter.

But this was different. This was panic, yes, but the panic was somehow a separate thing from the experience itself. It was like eating breakfast while listening to the radio: you can do either without concentrating on the other. I'm sure Nigella saw it differently, but in my head I felt as if I was concentrating on the experience rather than the panic.

I'd like to be able to tell you that I saw the great light before me, the smiling, beautiful people readying the blissful room to receive me, but I didn't. On the other hand just before I passed out, my feelings of tragic poignancy – a mixture of already missing Nigella and the children and feeling stupid at having

C

cancer but dying of this – were replaced by those of a warm calm. It was, I imagined, the sort of thing which drowning victims are meant to feel just after they've gone down for the third time.

The next thing I knew I was coming round with a mask over my face and some new tubes attached to me in the resuscitation room at the Charing Cross Hospital down the road in Fulham. They had wanted to give me a tracheotomy there and then; Nigella, mindful that portions of my neck and throat had just been rearranged by the country's top head and neck man, made the registrar get in touch with the Marsden, who got word to Rhŷs Evans who instructed that all other things being equal his people should be allowed to cut a new breathing hole in my throat.

Meanwhile I was breathing an oxygen-helium mixture and the gunky blockage had been cleared. There was some worry about the EEG reading: apparently when I'd reached the hospital my oxygen-starved heart was under such a strain there was a suspicion I was having a heart attack. But by the time Rhŷs Evans had been contacted and the Charing Cross people had agreed I could be taken by the Marsden I seemed to be OK.

That night we slept, but barely, on separate trolleys in the resuscitation room and at 9 a.m. the next day an ambulance, complete with flashing light and siren, rushed us round to the Marsden at the other end of the borough. I was put into a ward full of old men for a while and then transferred back into Room F, an old lag being welcomed back to his old cell.

In an hour the porter dropped in to move me down to the theatre for a rather more leisurely tracheotomy than the emergency job I might otherwise have had, and I realised that it held no fear for me at all. Just a year or so earlier I'd allowed the then unsuspected cancer to progress who-knows-how-much further because I was terrified of the idea of a general anaesthetic; here I was now, about to go under for the fifth time (cyst, biopsy, endoscopy, operation, tracheotomy) and thinking nothing of it. But then my reactions to so many things had changed over the months.

Take the pill, for instance.

The episode with the allergist all those years earlier took place while I was waiting for a referral to the stressed-out bastards department of Bart's Hospital. Not long after my 30th birthday I was lying in bed with my then wife, Anne-Marie, a woman who'd been a dance teacher in a school down the road from the one in which I taught drama. At 2 a.m. I woke Annie up screaming in panic: I was, I told her, having (a) a nervous breakdown and (b) a heart attack. I had no chest pain whatsoever, but I was convinced that my heart was giving out. It was the start of my subsequent fear of a heart attack.

This was in the days when family doctors would still come out at 2 a.m. Our man turned up, explained what a panic attack was and gave me a Valium to calm me. Until that moment I'd never had the slightest glimpse of what mental instability might look like, and the new possibilities terrified me. The next morning I turned up at his surgery and he offered me three choices. I could start on a course of sedatives in the hope that everything would go away; I could sign up with a psychiatric social worker; or I could be referred to the shrinks at Bart's. The first sounded dangerous: even then the dangers of Valium addiction were occasioning long articles in the Sunday papers. Psychiatric social work sounded a little low-rent – rather the thing I imagined they might offer teenage single mothers who'd threatened to jump off the top floor.

C

And so I was referred to Bart's where six months later I was put on the schedule of a psychotherapist. By this time I was working at London Weekend Television, a company with a culture so testosteronish that to have mentioned that I needed time off for therapy would have been to have asked for my cards. And so I agreed with the therapist that I'd be therapied at 8 a.m. each Friday morning.

I tried my hardest to be a good psychotherapeutic patient, but I couldn't do it. She'd turn up ten minutes late and ask me how I felt about her being ten minutes late and I'd say it's OK. She'd say wasn't I angry at her? And I'd say that, well, I imagined the bus didn't turn up: it happens. Eventually I understood that I was meant to get angry, but by the time realisation came she was the one who sat and glowered each week. Or I'd dig deep into my psyche and find something which sounded as if it might be useful about my potty training or my feelings for my brothers, except that I'd get carried away with the part I was playing of therapee and start to elaborate the stories beyond their possible outcome, and she'd glower at me some more.

Eventually I was handed over to the hospital's stress management unit, which was much more the thing, and after six months of that I was sent out into the world to find a therapist of my own.

My years in therapy finished when, a couple of years later, my man persuaded me that we had gone as far together as we were likely to and that what I should really do by way of a therapeutic coda was to turn up at a men's group he was running. This met on the top floor of a villa in Finsbury Park in North London which was given over entirely to various forms of therapy. As I climbed to the attic each week I could hear the rebirthers screaming on the ground floor, the Gestalt clients grunting as they beat their bean-bag mothers with plastic baseball bats on the first floor, the yogis om-ing on the floor above that.

On the top floor a dozen of us sat round in a softly lit beige room and talked about the experience of being a man.

I can't remember what happened on the first week, but on the second a chap asked us for our input with a problem he was having. As regulars knew, he said, he had a pretty full week of therapeutic activity. On Monday he had his intermediate sexuality class and on Tuesday he was doing group therapy. Wednesday was this, his men's group, and Thursday was his long-standing personal therapy session. And on Fridays he was heavily involved with the Gestalt group. The thing was, he said, his therapist had advised that he could usefully take part in a new self-awareness group which he was starting on Saturday afternoons. What did we all think?

We all thought that this sounded like an excellent way to spend a Saturday afternoon: what, after all, could be more useful than another couple of hours of worried introspection? It occurred to me that these weren't people in need of therapy but hobbyists who did therapy like other men went fishing or built model aeroplanes. The only difference was that this was rather more expensive.

But I thought it was unfair of me to drop the group on the basis of this single fatuousness. I went back the next week. This time another member wanted our input. This man was so big that when he waddled over and sat on a beige three-seat sofa there was no room for anybody else on it. He must have weighed well over 20 stone and how he got up to that attic room without suffering cardiac arrest I have no idea.

His problem was that he just could not get laid. He'd tried every way known of meeting girls, but none of them would sleep with him. What did we all think?

We all gave our ideas. Perhaps he wasn't being as honest with them as he might be; perhaps he could use the assertiveness training group which met on Mondays; perhaps a bright new tie would help. This went on for two hours and at no time during that period did anyone – me included – say that the problem might have anything to do with him weighing the same as his car. That was the last meeting I attended.

(In fact I wrote about the meetings a few years later in my *Times* column, and six weeks later got a pained letter from the group's leader and my ex-therapist. As I read the letter two things were apparent: (a) that most of the people who'd been in the group that night were still meeting together, their problems still unsettled and (b) that my column had been the subject of their meeting for the weeks in between its appearance and their drafting this letter.)

Whatever. I won't pretend that the few years of therapy weren't useful, not least because they staunched the panic attacks fairly soon after they started. But once I'd had the first attack and was aware that this temporary terror could strike at any time I started carrying around a few temazepam – a sedative generally used as a sleeping pill, and a Valium relative. Eventually the pills became the sort of psychopharmacological equivalent of a lucky rabbit's foot and a couple of chipped and flaking pills would sit in a little silver pill case for years without ever running the risk of being swallowed. Nonetheless, I always carried them with me and I had been known to turn round and drive home if, a mile down the road, I patted my trouser pockets and realised that the small lump wasn't there.

I'd been carrying the pill, and its successors, for, I guess, 14 years when Mady phoned that night. But now as I went down to the theatre again I was as pill-less as I had been for three or four months. Talismans seemed, nowadays, to be impotent in the face of real life. And in any case, here I was dealing with real life, unreal as it seemed.

There were times, I admit, when these sorts of personal and internal change tempted me to believe that the cancer was in some way a good thing. Readers would write and suggest that my apparent ability to face up to things wasn't just a silver lining to a nasty black cloud but that there was no cloud at all. There was. For whatever minor psychological benefits I may have been garnering from all this there was nothing of any use happening for Nigella or the children.

I came round from the operation with a plastic pipe poking out of my neck just above the top of my breastbone. The tube was below my vocal cords and so there was no way of getting puff from my lungs to them. I was dumb again.

The trachy – it turns out that we trachy-wearers call them this – was a four-inch arc of plastic tubing which fitted into the hole in my throat and down into my windpipe and was stopped from falling all the way in by a flange on the outer side which was held tight to my neck by a length of white cloth tape. According to the big trachy poster on the inside of the little procedures room off Weston Ward where trachies were changed and cleaned and generally played with, there were ten different tubes to choose from: mine was a cuffed, unfenestrated model. The cuff was a little balloon around the tube which could be pumped up to make a proper seal in my windpipe, and the lack of fenestration meant there wasn't a window in either the main tube or its inner tube.

All of which is rather more than you need to know about trachy

C

tubes other than that they hurt like hell at first and need a lot of looking after in rather the way I imagine false teeth need looking after.

But it wasn't the pain or the hygiene regime which worried me but the fact of the trachy itself. I'd been warned that I might come round from the operation with tracheotomy and gastrectomy tubes already in place: that I hadn't done so meant a lot to me. I was ahead of the odds. But finding myself back on par again was somehow worse than having been given the tube during the operation. I had failed in some way.

Chapter 10

C

As if to make up for the illicit time off I'd been allowed at the end of my last visit I was kept in hospital for four nights. Most of the nurses were, for the best reasons, sorry enough to see me back: while there were a couple whose raised eyebrows suggested that they'd told me this was just what happens when naughty little boys go home early, most of them had rightly seen my early departure as a reflection on their skills as much as on my fortitude.

Just before I left this time round they swapped my tube for one which allowed me to speak – a term which I use, you understand, in its very loosest sense. A little plastic valve fitted over the end of the tube and blocked off the airway when I was breathing out, allowing the air to pass through my vocal cords. The tube clicked and gasped with the valve on and any listener had to be particularly well motivated to understand anything I might try and say. Over the tube I wore a Buchanan Bib – a cross between a cravat and a string vest, soaked in water to humidify the tube and opaque to protect the sensibilities of a public which doesn't like to see its fellows walking around with gaping holes in their necks.

The nurses loaded me with the gear I'd need as a trachy-man – brushes, sponge pads, spare tapes – and sent me home.

Nigella was looking after the kids and would be coming to pick me up at 6 p.m. but I was ready earlier: I decided to hail a cab on the Fulham Road just as if I were an ordinary person. Happily there was one which had just set down outside the hospital as I left.

'Where to?' he said.

I tried to give my address but even with my new valve it came out as a series of honks and clicks. No matter: I was realistic. I'd written down the address against just such an eventuality. I

C

started patting my pockets, looking for the note I'd made, honking and dribbling my unintelligible glossectomee's version of 'Hold on' and 'I know I've got it here somewhere'. The cabby looked upset and uncomfortable: I don't know what association he made with my lack of voice but he obviously thought it connected with the pantomime I was going through as I searched for the piece of paper. Eventually I found it and showed it to him and we started off in silence.

The meter read eight pounds when we got home: I handed over a ten-pound note.

'No,' he said, and started to put the cab into gear.

I honked and waved the tenner at him.

'No. I don't want it.'

He looked at me miserably. This was his act of charity. I threw the money down next to his seat. He picked it up, came round and pushed it into one of the carrier bags I was holding.

'No,' he said again, and drove off, angry with my ungraciousness.

Here I was, hale apart from the small portion between my nose and my neck, earning a living, cabbing it to a reasonable home in a reasonable part of town. And what did he see? I really don't know. A man coming home from the cancer ward to die? A mute who, by that definition alone, must need the money?

There had been some depressing moments in those months but none quite so depressing as standing on the pavement watching the cabby drive away without my money, pitying me for an illness I didn't have.

The two carrier bags into which the cabby had tried to stuff my money were marked PATIENT'S PROPERTY in a rather dodgy Wormwood Scrubs sort of way, and contained my latest collection of cancer victim takeaway gear.

It had now been some five months since I'd been diagnosed as having cancer and slightly longer since I had the first operation and was sent home with a grimace and a bottle of painkillers. In the interim I seemed to have collected a small pharmacy and as I threw my latest collection on top of the pile, I took stock.

So far BUPA had bought me:

Four boxes co-proxamol (paracetamol and codeine painkillers);

Four boxes co-codamol (ditto, more or less);

Two large cartons co-codamol dispersible (or soluble to you and me, for the period just after the operation when I couldn't swallow pills);

Two bottles Voltarol (heavy-duty painkiller usually given to mothers *post partum*; big advantage is that can be taken at the same time as the paracetamol preparations without overdosing. By working out timings and interactions carefully it's possible to take three different painkillers, each marked 'To be taken every six hours' every two hours. It's what we in the suffering business call 'pain management');

Three boxes dispersible Voltarol, raspberry flavoured. Why raspberry? Why not?

One bottle diclofenac. The generic name for Volterol.

One bottle Zantac. Was a treatment for stomach ulcers until they discovered stomach ulcers are caused by a bug. Now used to mollify potential stomach problems caused by Volterol;

Three bottles temazepam. Sedative masquerading as sleeping pill. Bottles almost full. To my amazement haven't felt the need for sedatives and in their sleeping pill guise they don't work against my wakeful epiglottis. Who'd have thought I'd ever have the need to write a sentence which included the words 'my wakeful epiglottis'?

C

One bottle temazepam elixir. Drinkable sleeping pills;

One bottle lactulose. Laxative for those living on the mmmmm! so-tasty Jevity diet;

Six assorted tracheotomy tubes, plus assorted inner tubes, introduction tubes, blanking plugs and other accessories for the fashionable tracheostomee about town;

Two tubes of KY jelly for sliding tracheotomy tube into the hole in my throat;

Three tracheotomy brushes for cleaning what the nurses delicately call 'secretions' from the tube. Said secretions vary from light covering of phlegm to chunks of hard, brown nastiness cementing the tube to the hairs on my chest. Who'd be a nurse?

One bottle Hydrex. Dangerous pink disinfectant in which tracheotomy brushes are stored;

One bottle cyclizine hydrochloride. Anti-emetic to stop sickness during radiotherapy;

Two bottles metoclopramide. As above, but effective.

One bottle metoclopramide hydrochloride solution. As above but for non-pill-swallowers.

One box co-danthramer capsules. Laxative to overcome constipation caused by morphine.

One bottle amitriptyline hydrochloride. Normally prescribed as an antidepressant, but also has painkilling function. Stopped using it when discovered also has a beating over head with sock full of sand and feel like a zombie for half the day function.

Two large boxes Lyofoam. Sponge pads which sit between the flange of the tracheotomy and the neck to soak up secretions. Have two boxes because accidentally prescribed Lyofoam Red instead of Lyofoam Green. Lyofoam Red lacks hole for tracheotomy. We trachy-types know these things.

C

100 six-inch-long cotton buds in sterile wraps. Used for removing secretions from between tracheotomy and chest.

Twelve disposable forceps. Used for picking the chunkier secretions off.

Two bottles Corsodyl Mint for swabbing round mouth and tongue in act of oral hygiene, now that I live a life where men in white coats regularly ask questions like 'So how's our oral hygiene at the moment?'

Two packs 50 octagonal sponge pads on sticks for sluicing Corsodyl around mouth.

Sundry Buchanan bibs and the like from a company in Leeds which specialises in accoutrements for laryngectomees and tracheyostomees.

100 swabs for holding my tongue with. For the life of me I can't remember why I had to do this.

Four syringes of Instillagel antiseptic lignocaine. The ulcer-numbing gel which I used to such effect on *Newsnight*.

Eight plastic syringes, various. These were left over from the period just after my first homecoming when I had to inject antibiotics and dispersible painkillers into my feeding tube.

Four antibiotics, various. All now empty and so only in my pharmacy in spirit.

Six orange rubber and glass atomiser sprays for keeping my tracheotomy moist now that the trachea wasn't being bathed in the warm and humid air which comes, oral hygiene permitting, from my mouth.

Six Durogesic 25. The morphine equivalent of the nicotine patch: stick them to somewhere non-hairy and watch them leak morphia into the body for three days. Yowza!

Six Durogesic 50. As above, but double strength.

One box assorted tapes, wipes, syringes, plasters, dressings,

C

creams, lotions, disposable scissors, forceps. Donated to the Diamond surgical archive from time to time and not yet catalogued.

In fact the amount of this rubbish I needed at any one time was rarely in proportion to my condition. Not long after the operation when, by most standards, I was at my illest I needed very few drugs and no hardware. A couple of weeks later, when the swelling was going down and the scar tissue was forming, I was much nearer to good health but stuck on a rota of four different painkillers a day. The tracheostomy brought with it a whole new set of apparatus and lotions and required me to demonstrate an attention to routine which I just couldn't muster.

But the greatest quantities of traffic from the Marsden pharmacy were stored in the kitchen rather than in the bathroom.

I had watched my weight fall gradually from the start of the radiotherapy. At first, as I say, I assumed the loss was entirely due to my eating less; in fact it had much more to do with the tumour. People with cancer lose weight. But now with the golf ball removed I was nominally tumour free and I needed to start putting some weight on – both because I needed some substance in order for the operative wounds to heal and also to prove to myself that there wasn't some undiscovered tumour still eating away at me.

But my weight was dropping. Each week Nigella would report to my new dietitian, Sam White, on what I'd eaten recently and Sam would explain that it wasn't quite enough.

By now I'd stopped hooking myself up to the Jevity bottle, had the tube removed from my nose and was back on my old radiotherapy diet of Build-Up and Ready-Brek. The difference

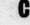

this time was that not only had I lost my sense of taste, but that my throat wouldn't allow anything but liquids to pass. It meant I had to swallow at least 2,000 liquid calories a day, which translated as either eight Build-Ups or half that many Scandishakes, another powdered nutrient which came from the hospital pharmacy rather than from Boots' shelves. Whatever: they were, at best, simply maintaining my weight.

I had transcended the stage I hit during the first radiotherapy course where I became a person stuck at his proper weight: I had become a thin person. When I told people that I was not quite myself I meant it almost literally: in the mirror I was somebody else. Precisely, I was a little old man whom I imagined to be called Albert or Norman or George.

Certainly I was little, or at least littler than I ever have been in my adult life. This wasn't ordinary weight loss – the few pounds you can't face hanging over the top of your bathing trunks, or the wobbly stone that lingers *post partum*, but real missing weight, whole chunks of corporation, enough spare body to make another small person. By my reckoning, I had lost a leg and a half's worth of me.

And it was an old leg and a half's worth, at that: a leg and a half's worth from the days when my thigh still had its familiar triangular cross-section and my calf bulged over the top of my sock. Now I looked in the mirror and saw a different man looking back, a stranger whose stick legs dropped away from his tiny rump, whose wiry arms were only muscle and bone and ropey vein, a man with very little belly to speak of. I had the new age body that I always associated with the sort of men who dress in draw-string trousers, run primal scream therapy sessions in North London and tell you that they've never felt healthier since they went fruitarian in '87. I couldn't tell the time because the

C

now oversize metal bracelet on my watch allowed the face to swing round to the wrong side of my wrist and Nigella had to buy me a second, smaller, wedding ring to stop the original one, which had once been tight, from falling off.

It meant that for the first time in my life I could share jeans with my partner. Ever since I was a teenager I've thought there was something ineffably cool about men sharing clothes with their partners. I mean, not tights or stilettos, of course, but as a child of tubbiness I always envied those men who would bound out of the college halls of residence in the morning in their girlfriends' Levis.

But wearing Nigella's hipsters was the full extent of my new youthfulness. My new little old manliness had nothing to do with age or even with deterioration, but with my own bodily frailty and the state of my bedroom and bathroom and office, all of which were littered with the little-old-man impedimenta of my new medical routines. The things I had to do each day with orange rubber bulbs, and special stiff brushes dripping pungent pink cleaning fluids were the sort of things that little old men have to do. Three times a day I pottered around the bathroom squeezing bulbs, and cleaning tubes and sluicing parts of my body out and taking pills against pain and swelling and infection.

And as so many of my correspondents were keen to remind me, however sympathetically, hardly any of my squeezing and sluicing or the symptoms which occasioned them had anything to do with the cancer. They were all the product of the cure for cancer ('cure' being a word which all too often they put in quotation marks so as to show how hollow they thought the concept to be). This was iatrogenic illness: illness caused by doctors.

They were right. Iatrogenic illness was just what it was. And there were times when I had to remind myself that it was the iatrogenic illness which was saving my life. The more mealy-mouthed alternativist always suggested there was no difference between a patient suffering the honest iatrogenic illness caused by excising a tumour and, say, the patient who is felled by one of the nasty bugs that inhabit certain hospitals, or the patient who suffers at the hands of an incompetent doctor. Angry as I got with the fact of my cancer and the symptoms of its cure, I never doubted that the alternative to those symptoms was early death.

Nonetheless, in one of those moments of anger and not long after I made a list of the contents of my new medicine cabinet, I wrote a note in my diary listing my current symptoms. Almost a month after the main operation it read:

1. Frozen right shoulder where neck dissection sliced through nerves and muscle. Left hand now extends six inches further above my head than right.

2. Shooting pains in neck and jaw as post-operative numbness wears off and scar tissue starts to build up.

3. Constant bad earache as result of referred pain from scar at back of tongue.

4. Missing saliva glands on left-hand side of throat and part of tongue. (The next lot of radiotherapy would deal with most of the rest of the saliva glands.)

5. Small bald patch at back of head just below larger, natural bald patch.

6. Temporary – I hoped – loss of taste-buds accompanied by burning sensation on tongue when eating food with any taste at all.

7. Slight limp. I'm still not quite sure what caused this but I

C

realised not long after I left the Marsden that I couldn't lift my right foot properly. Worried that the radiotherapy might have hit my spinal column by mistake I was sent off to the National Neurological Hospital in Bloomsbury when a genial man spent an afternoon giving me electric shocks. The best guess of all parties was that I was leant on fairly heavily while under the anaesthetic and that this caused a nerve to be trapped.

8. Oedema around neck and chin. On the one hand all the lymph nodes in the area had been taken away, on the other there was now a series of scars which, between them, connected me ear to ear. It would be some months before the various fluids which were hanging around in my new dewlaps would find an escape route.

9. Missing beard on right-hand side of face, the result of radiotherapy.

10. Overproduction of mucus.

11. Overproduction of saliva.

12. Various ulcers around the original radiotherapy site.

13. Sore back. For the most part this was because I'd lost all the fatty padding from around the area, leaving the vertebrae unprotected, and had yet to find a new sleeping position.

14. Impossibly sore throat.

15. Toothache. When I was booked for my second lot of radiotherapy Sarah Howells took out another tooth directly above the one I'd lost on the first round. Apart from the soreness of the toothless gum, the gum below the adjoining healthy teeth had dropped back very slightly leaving me horribly susceptible to pain from hot or cold foods.

16. A rackety and painful night-time cough caused by the mucus and extra saliva slithering down the wrong hole and into my bruised windpipe.

17. At any given time, and depending on the nature of my diet that week, either chronic constipation or chronic diarrhoea.
18. Missing lump of tongue.

I wasn't sure whether the missing tongue counted as iatrogenic: it had, after all, contained the tumour. But as far as some of my correspondents were concerned, even allowing the tumour to be removed showed a dangerous willingness on my part to subjugate myself to medical orthodoxy. Just before the big operation I'd been at a party where a weasel-faced man with a ponytail made a point of bumping into me so that he could tell me that he didn't know why I was making so much fuss about the cancer.

'It is,' he said, not bothering to stretch further than necessary for his cliché, 'all in the mind.' Well not *all*, perhaps, and he was willing to grant that when the oafs who call themselves doctors looked down their so-called microscopes they might have seen something which they called, in that cynical and arbitrary way doctors have, cancer, but that was, he said, to miss his point.

The thing was that whatever I chose to call my dis-ease (he split the syllables and hardened the first 's' because he is the first to have worked out the subtle etymology of the word 'disease') whether I was cured or not was a matter for me to decide. If I got my head right, got my energy levels sorted out, fought the disease in my soul, then I'd kick it. He didn't actually use the words 'vibes' or 'chakra' but it was a pretty close thing.

There was also something about some medical regime practised in Vietnam which was absolutely guaranteed to deal with all nasty western diseases, and stupidly I went for that and asked him why it is that all the best medical systems from the mystic East and deepest Africa come from countries where the average lifespan is that of a World War I pilot with a death wish. (In fact I've since checked: the average male in Vietnam lives only ten fewer years than his British equivalent and I imagine that as he lies dying in middle age he thanks his god that he doesn't have to suffer all that dangerous and imprecise western medicine.)

Ponytail ker-chawed and pointed out that longevity is not a valid measure of national healthiness, and I said that oddly enough it was one which had always worked for me, and we sort of left it at that which was probably just as well because had I tackled him on the question of whose responsibility my cancer is I'd have got angry and he'd have told me about stress levels and I'd have kicked him hard in the chakras, knocking several of his energy meridians severely out of kilter.

'It seems,' I wrote in *The Times* that week, 'that there is a small space where new age philosophy meets sharp-heeled Thatcherism and it is in the idea that we are all entirely responsible for our individual physical states. In a way, of course, that's true enough: my choice to smoke for all those years, to live in the centre of our smokiest city, to eat full English breakfasts in bad provincial hotels must certainly have taken its toll on heart and artery and bronchial tube.

'And yes, if I still smoked and carried on doing so through the treatment I would accept that I may bear the responsibility for the cure not working. It's the idea of taking spiritual responsibility for a disease once it's been diagnosed which annoys me. For it leads to the idea of the survivor as personal hero – that only those who want to survive enough get through to the end, and the implied corollary that those who die are somehow lacking in moral fibre and the will to live.

'I'll accept that some can grit their teeth and get through the treatments more happily than others, and even that there are various calming regimes which make the treatment slightly more bearable. In terms of responsibility, though, as far as I'm concerned I will be cured only if the surgeons have cut out the right bits of my neck and the radiologists and radiographers have chosen the right bits of my throat to point their machine at.'

In fact, by now the radiologists had found a new place to point their machines at. I'd been back to the Marsden for a new mask to be made up and a new set of interior images to be created on the simulator, and the radiographers in both departments greeted me with a small, tight-lipped, sorry-to-see-you-back smile. Until the final few depressing days of the last 30 sessions I'd usually come into the room with a smile and a joke, and the radiographers usually returned the favour. This time, though, it was different. I would give my own tight-lipped smile each day, strip off my top and heave my shrunken body on to the bench, without a joke or even much of a greeting. Occasionally I'd have a radiotherapist who hadn't been around during my last sessions and who insisted on instructing me in the way of the irradiating wave. I wanted to tell them that I'd now been smacked on the neck with irradiation 40 or 50 or whatever times, thanks all the same, but it was too much effort, and so I would just glower at them.

True, last time all my tongue was still there and it was easier to joke, but this time we all seemed to understand that the odds had changed.

Changing odds must be the unchanging condition at the Marsden. For so long now one of the thoughts which had sustained me was that however terrible a state some of the people I saw at the hospital looked to be in, somebody here, somebody who knew about cancer reckoned it worth their while trying to find the right treatment. The prematurely and artificially bald man who could only move to the radiotherapy room by clinging to his wife's shoulders and moving in tiny, painfully slow steps: somebody thought it worth giving him radiotherapy. The wan, stick-thin woman glimpsed in one of the day wards on the ground floor: somebody who knew what they were talking about had decided that it was worth carrying on shooting her body full of toxic, but possibly life-saving, drugs. It must be, I reasoned, that these peope have a chance of living. The sustaining corollary, of course, was that if they had a chance in their state, then my chances as a patient able to drive himself round to the hospital, must be somewhat better.

But as we swapped painful smiles on my first day back in the radiotherapy suite and one of the radiologists said 'Sorry to see you back. I didn't expect you to be one of the returners', I understood how often the staff here must see somebody turn up for their first treatment unscarred, full of life and substance, and return again and again, each time less vital, less hopeful, each time the odds slightly lower.

One day at breakfast Cosima turned to me and smiled. 'You're going to die, Daddy.' It struck me as the most appallingly tasteless prediction I could imagine and I flew into one of the rages that were becoming too common. Cosima was three and a half, had no idea what death means or what my illness was. It turned out that she'd overheard her nanny telling a friend on the phone that on the night of my near-death experience she thought I was going to die.

I went and found Cosima and apologised to her. She said, 'I

can't remember a time when you could speak properly', and I knew how she felt.

Meanwhile I had started speech therapy.

In the head and neck game, speech therapy means rather more than just teaching people how to speak again, and in particular it's concerned with teaching them how to eat. I was swallowing no better now than I had been in hospital. My own saliva was still collecting in pools at the front of my mouth and every so often I'd have to find a paper tissue and blow my mouth as others blow their nose. In my office and bedroom the waste baskets overflowed with soggy tissues. I could drink, yes, but whenever I drank anything it was impossible to get rid of the last mouthful. Indeed, the only way of getting anything down my throat was by using the next mouthful to push it down. In practice this meant that everything had to be eaten in one quick series of gulps and swallows lest I lose the momentum.

Not long after this, for instance, I had my very first post-operative outing and went with Bywater to the Groucho Club in Soho. I'd not had anything to drink for a few months now – and I mean drink as in *drink* – but I thought that a small whiskey diluted heavily with water shouldn't hurt my crippled tongue too much.

We sat in the upstairs bar and I took a sip of whiskey and rolled it round my mouth while I decided what to do next. Bywater asked a question. I answered. Of course I answered: if there was nothing else I knew how to do then I was an expert at sitting in the Groucho and swapping *bons mots*. As I answered the question, the mouthful of whiskey fell down my jacket front. Why would it not? I couldn't get it to the back of my throat without taking another mouthful and then the second mouthful would be left there. In the end I had three whiskeys by dint of putting each of them down my throat in one go and rushing to the lavatories to spit out the last, unswallowable, mouthful.

At home I had, at least, the advantage of not having to run to do my spitting in private, although I tried to keep the more dramatic hawking for when Cosima wasn't around.

Now that I was trying to get past the liquid stage, eating had become a pretty disgusting spectacle. I would take a swallow or a bite of something and, half the time, immediately start coughing. Bits of food would fly out of my mouth and nose. Sometimes the food would stay away from the sensitive areas at the back of my throat and I'd manage to get a bowl of muesli or crème caramel down my throat. Except, of course, for the last mouthful, which would stay there, unswallowed, for as long as I left it. I would wander over to the kitchen sink and spit out the last chunk of food, and then spit again to get out the particles dotted around my mouth, then take a swig of warm water – if it was too cold it hurt my teeth – and try and collect the lost food before taking a third swig.

It was the food's stagnancy which I found the most monstrous of all, I think. I would eat something, and brush my teeth, and then four hours later find myself hurled into a 20-minute coughing fit as some crumb or another decided eventually to dislodge itself from the crevice in which it had been hiding and sit on some scar tissue. My unmoving tongue meant that the only way I could clear debris from the roof of my mouth was with a finger or a brush; if I forgot who I now was for a couple of hours it would pile up in there in little layers like geological samples.

(I know: gross. What were you expecting when you bought a book on cancer?)

I was, understandably enough, not on everyone's dinner party list. But I was making some small progress. My biggest and most cheering postbag since the start of the cancer columns came when I wrote that I'd forced myself to stand over the sink and swallow a pear, chunk by chunk.

I was standing at the sink, about to spit a mouthful of baby pear down the waste-disposal, when I thought: no. I shall swallow this pear. I have not eaten a fruit in its true fruitful form since June – the vestigial lemon 'n' lime in the lemon 'n' lime Build-Up drinks on which I've subsisted for the past couple of months not counting – and I shall eat this one.

I almost did, too.

And as I almost got it all down my throat I thought, in one of those tearful moments of mad joy I have from time to time nowadays, how easy it's all been.

I'll start with the pear, because that's the quick bit, and then I'll go on to the easy life because I haven't decided yet whether or not that's one of the written thoughts which goes off for publication.

As you will know, constant reader, they took the back of my tongue out in June, leaving me unable to talk in any meaningful way for a while, although the exact definition of the term 'a while' is still in some dispute. What I wasn't expecting was the effect the new compact tongue – combined, it has to be said, with a second six-week stint of throat-burning radiotherapy – would have on my eating. Who knew the part the tongue played in this sort of thing?

Before I was forced to think about it I'd assumed you put the food in your mouth, chewed it about a bit, swallowed, moved on to the peas. It turns out that unless you have a fully functioning

C

tongue shovelling the stuff back towards the gullet as it passes through the scything teeth, the food just stays there at the front of your mouth, or worse, starts leaking back in the direction of the plate.

Hence the liquidity of my diet these few months past. But it's been two weeks since the radiotherapy stopped and they're talking about taking the tracheotomy tube out of my throat some time soon, and I thought I'd try something solid. Last night I started with a pint of Murphy's which occupies that pleasant intermediate state between liquid and solid and was the first alcohol I've touched since May. And then I tried some venison stew of which I managed that part of a single mouthful which didn't fall into the glass of Murphy's as I was trying to swig it down. That the rest of the stew finished up on the floor was through no fault of my tongue and entirely down to one of the rages I go into from time to time when not being me gets a little too much to bear.

And so tonight I tried a small, soft pear.

Same thing: chew, chew, dribble. The pear was about to go the way of the stew when I thought damn this thing, and made it go down my throat. It wasn't exactly Robert the Bruce, but I jumped a little and ran to tell everyone that I'd eaten a pear.

Which is when I realised that if I was going to eat and talk again I'd have to make myself do this time after time, day after day, and the extent to which I've lived a life where, thus far, I've been able to avoid doing most of the things I didn't want to do. Or, rather, wanted to have done but didn't want to do at that moment.

I didn't work at school and true, I didn't achieve what you'd call academic success, but I managed to find a good college where they appreciated certain sorts of academic failure. I didn't work overhard in the job I trained for, but managed to fluke my way into journalism at just the point where I could avoid a traditional tedious training full of shorthand and typing. I screwed up a first marriage through indolence, although not that alone, and lucked myself into a second one with the right wife who had the secret of manufacturing perfect kids. Who could have my luck?

And then all this happened – and even then I've not been in a position to decide between the easy and the hard hauls: hard as the illness has been it has been one without choices.

But here I stand at the sink with strands of pear juice running down my chin, and I know I have to force myself to do this every day until I can do it as easily as you can do it, and for some reason it makes me unreasonably happy.

At the Marsden the main speech therapist charged with helping me though this was away for a couple of weeks and I was given over to a New Zealander on temporary attachment to the hospital. She sat me down and took me through a questionnaire. Was I drinking this, eating that, swallowing the other? What happened if I drank the other or ate this?

I told her about the coughing and my inability to polish off the last mouthful of anything and she gave me a blank smile. Her worry was that if I was so unable to control my food some of it would go down the wrong hole and...

And what? I'd drown? I thought not. Everything which was going down the wrong way seemed to find its way back up again quite happily. Even so, she said, she was banning thin liquids. Thin liquids included water, tea, coffee, beer. True, I'd not had a beer for a while, but I was looking forward to one some day and meanwhile I certainly wasn't giving up water. Nor would she if her saliva had the consistency of sump oil. She gave me another blank little smile.

C

Eventually she fixed me up with a video swallow. In a dank little room in the basement of the Marsden I took a swig of something that would show up on an X-ray and then swallowed it while the X-ray machine glowed and a video camera recorded the swig's progress down my throat. The consultant overseeing the swallow looked pleased enough: there was a tiny amount of fluid going over the edge and into the windpipe but, as he said, 'There's probably more leakage in my own throat. It looks fine.'

The speech therapist disagreed. Even a tiny amount like this could be dangerous. There was no question of her balancing the minute chance of my doing any serious harm against the immense relief the water brought: her ban stayed. So I ignored it. The alternativists who wrote to me at *The Times* were always telling me that alternative medicine was about seizing control of one's illness. Well, this was me seizing control of mine. I decided that I'd go to Stephanie Kingham, the ex-Marsden therapist who had phoned me just before the operation, to learn how to speak again.

Chapter 11

C

Friends would tell me differently, but as far as I was concerned, my voice was not improving. And just as my missing taste-buds had continued to surprise me every time I put food in my mouth and found as if for the first time that it had no taste, so was I continually surprised by what came out of my mouth when I opened it to speak. In the milliseconds before I spoke I would hear the words in my head, sounding quite normal, very John Diamond, and I'd open my mouth to say them and what would come out would be somebody doing that honking impression of Charles Laughton in a bubbly, underwater version of *The Hunchback of Notre Dame* rendered doubly liquid when, as often as not, the reservoir of saliva which had gathered at the front would start to leak out by the thought's third word. I was forever speaking through the corner of my handkerchief like a dandy in a bad Reformation comedy.

And so I would start to ask people for things in shops, because that is what I am used to doing, and I'd get two words into the sentence before I'd realise that neither of us was going to get to the other end of it unscathed. Or there was the Saturday when out on a credit-card sabotaging mission I turned into a street opposite Selfridge's which was being wilfully blocked by a BT cable-laying van, and when the man wouldn't move it I started having a row with him, just as if I was somebody who could have loud rows in the street. Which, it turns out, one can't when the only thing the person you're trying to have a row with says is 'Sorry? What? No I can't understand...' and then, when he gets bored with your honking, impenetrable voice, tells you to piss off.

It wasn't much different with those who had attuned themselves to my honking: each had a different way of not understanding me. Some would just look blankly, running over

C

the sounds in their head hoping they could unscramble them in retrospect and then when I was halfway through the next sentence say 'No, sorry, didn't get it.' Others would nod enthusiastically whatever I'd say in the apparent belief that if they got two out of every three words they'd have a vague idea what I was on about. Occasionally I'd slip them a series of meaningless honks and add 'don't you?' at the end, and they'd answer with an even bigger nod. Which would have been a fine gag except that its implications depressed me more than it made a point to whoever I was talking to.

The only two people to understand me regardless, or, at least, to have found a way of saying 'what?' in the way one says it when one doesn't catch something in the course of normal conversation, were Nigella and Cheryl, who came in to help Nigella from time to time and who, over the months, became something of a life-saver, filling in when nannies resigned, when we suddenly needed, the two of us, to get away from the house and the children for a couple of hours, when the mess had exploded about us and we needed setting to rights.

But just as I forgot what my new voice was like there was a transitional point when I realised I'd forgotten what the old one sounded like too. One midweek day I switched the car radio on halfway through that lunchtime slot when Radio 4 goes all jocular, and there was a quartet of standard issue Radio 4 panellists solving droll crossword clues for a chuckling Broadcasting House theatre audience.

I'd missed the introductions, but I could work out who a couple of the panellists were, given how often their voices turn up on the sort of shows where you have to solve crossword clues, or know what Clem Atlee so famously said to Bessie Braddock on Derby Day in 1948, or for two points per ingredient, guess the contents of this fascinating medieval recipe for quince syllabub, but I couldn't put a name to the others – even though one seemed vaguely familiar. His was a deepish voice, southern, with a very slight cynical lisp and a...

Hold on, though. It was me. It was a programme I'd recorded in a pre-operative era when I still had all of a tongue and could rent it out for lisping and cynical purposes.

Coming unexpectedly upon my pre-cancerous self like that was like looking from the cold station platform into a brightly lit and crowded train and seeing the twin brother I'd forgotten I had idly turning the page of his paper. Twin, but not identically so, because the other odd thing was the potency of my sense of the me listening being a different me from the me on the radio. I heard a different voice but my experience in that split second of realisation was of a whole different life. And strangely I was most conscious of *his* lack of realisation of the difference between the two lives. He was the one who didn't realise what a boon an unimpaired voice was, who ate his food without stopping to think about its remarkable flavour, who was criminally profligate with words, who took his wife and children and friends for granted – in short who didn't know he was living. And a man, at that, who had the appalling possibilities of life pegged so terribly wrongly. For the John Diamond on the radio the worst was the mundane death or madness which had threatened him all those years ago in the guise of a panic attack. What little imagination he had!

But if the man on the radio was unimaginative and ignorant, at least his *doppelgänger* listening in the car had become quite the metaphysician and knew all of those things now. I was still unwilling to acknowledge that I was better for knowing them because the knowledge cut both ways and carried, as far as I was concerned, many more cons than it did pros. What's more, the real question was whether I'd acquired that knowledge too late to be of much use.

But some of this was going to change – in vocal terms, at least. I had Stephanie the speech therapist, a wonderful woman with the voice of one who does the continuity announcements for some heavenly radio station, and who would teach me how to speak again.

She had her main practice in Dorking, but once or twice a week while Peter Rhŷs Evans was in a surgery somewhere sawing bones she would take over his rooms in Harley Street.

For all that I was still refusing to see silver linings, there was something rather attractive about getting a second chance at one of the basic psycho-social skills, not least because there was part of me which felt like a be-stumped Douglas Bader saying to the prosthetics people: 'Look, as long as you're popping down to the leg stores anyway you might as well make me 6'3'''. In the same way I wanted to tell Stephanie that while we were rebuilding the rubble of my voice in the hope that I could start broadcasting again in the autumn, I'd quite like this time round to be Alvar Liddell or Brian Perkins rather than the bloke with the North London lisp.

Nigella, who'd done Chomsky to a crisp at Oxford, thought the whole idea of studying one's own voice in order to recreate it for a second time was fascinating, and I too might have been fascinated had this been a theoretical rather than an abstruse practical problem.

The procedure looked simple enough. I would turn up at Harley Street once a week, usually with Nigella, and the three of us would sit around and talk for ten minutes or so, apparently just for the sake of it. And then Stephanie would make me repeat something I'd said in conversation and we'd all inspect the quality of my sibilants or the colour of my fricatives. I'd repeat some lists of meaningless sentences tuned to build up skills in particular parts of the tongue, chat some more, do some more repetitions. At the end of the hour my tongue and throat hurt in the way my biceps might have hurt if I'd done an hour's weight training.

It all took so *long*. From where I was sitting I was making no progress at all because every time I opened my mouth I gave myself the same implicit goal – to sound like me – and every time I failed. Worse, the therapy itself was terribly hard work, all that tah-tah-taying in front of the mirror and building up the discrete little muscles that I'd never been aware of before. It might have been easier if I were starting from scratch, like my son Bruno, but like a man taking driving lessons who has already been driving unlicensed through the back streets for years I already had too many bad habits to be broken. I knew, for instance, how to speak fast, but fast was the last thing Stephanie wanted me to speak. And so she would force me to slow everything down, to sound like a badly acted Eliza Doolittle in the first post-elocution conversation scene in *Pygmalion*. It was bad enough having a wonky voice but having a wonky voice and sounding like a stupid person was intolerable.

At the end of October I faxed Grizzie Burgess, my broadcast agent, and told her the reason I was faxing her was because if I phoned she wouldn't understand a word I was saying and for that reason alone she should get in touch with *People's Parliament* and *Fourth Column* and tell them that I wasn't a broadcaster again yet.

This was depressing news for all sorts of reasons – because *Fourth Column* was being dropped in the latest round of Radio 4

C

remakes and I would have liked to have done the last series, because dropping out of contracted work is never a good idea.

Worst of all, though, it made me reconsider the possibilities of my new life.

One afternoon Jemima Harrison was recording some meandering thought or another of mine for the TV.

'It's amazing how far you've come,' she said. 'Listen.'

And she played me back 30 seconds of my speech before I made her stop.

I knew that when we started the recordings after the operation I was all but incomprehensible and that if that footage was ever to be used it would have to be with subtitles. And I knew that in the past couple of weeks I had less often to repeat myself to make myself understood to friends who were tuned into my honk. But this was the first time I'd heard my voice since it stopped being my voice.

Do you remember how it was the first time you ever heard your own voice coming out of a tape recorder? How horrified you were that what sounded inside your head like a perfectly reasonable voice turned out to have been the trebly, breathy sound which came out of the loudspeaker? Well what I heard was that times ten. Until then I hadn't let myself realise that my voice was not just that of a man with a crippled throat but of one who was obviously insufficient elsewhere. I sounded, literally, disabled.

Fine: the world is full of disabled people who just get on with their lives more or less cheerfully, more or less resentfully, and I'm not going to tell you that they are less sensitive to their situation than I was at that moment to mine. But as I heard my voice I felt embarrassed to have been throwing it around the place unhindered for all this time. What could I have been thinking of? Of course that thought is, itself, embarrassing, but that's the sort of paradox which comes of writing this stuff down.

The other thing I knew in that moment was not only that there was no chance of my broadcasting again for a few months, but that there never had been such a chance. I knew how far my voice had progressed from the unintelligible honk I had when they took the breathing tube out to the point where I could make myself understood much of the time, and I knew how unlikely it was that anyone's voice could have progressed much further from that point in that time. True, I'd had the tracheotomy and was in the middle of the second radiotherapy course but those would only have set me back a few weeks at most and I was certainly more than a few weeks short of a broadcasting voice.

A couple of days later I put this to Rhŷs Evans, who nodded blandly and talked about the value of having the goal as opposed to that of achieving it, and I suppose I would have been more angry with the cheat which had been perpetrated if I had tried harder and spent more time tah-tah-taying at home.

Meanwhile the old routine had cranked up again: radiotherapy once a day, Rhŷs Evans once a week to have my throat felt, my scars inspected, my mouth prodded; Henk for much the same but from a radiological point of view.

At the start of the radiotherapy Henk talked about my cancer in a way which suggested that the labs still held remnants of it on file.

'Could I see it, then?' I said.

'See what?' said Henk.

'The slides with the sections of my cancer on them. Can I see them?'

Henk looked like a man demonstrating the dictionary

C

definition of being bemused. He blinked, he scratched his head, he started to talk and then stopped and then started again. He had, he said, been doing this for 25 years and in that time nobody had ever asked him if they could see their cancer.

I found this remarkable. I understood, of course, that I had made something of a fetish of my own cancer; it was part of the same process which led me to write about it so often, in that by rendering the cancer an objective spectacle I could distance myself from it. I remembered that on the first night Bywater had come round and led me through the Internet coverage of cancer I had downloaded a blown-up photograph of a squamous cell cancer of the neck which I'd found on some cancer site or another, and for some days used it as the background picture on my computer's desk top. And I knew that when, at the end of my first course of radiotherapy and when I still thought it would be my only course of radiotherapy, I asked to take the mask home with me, I'd got some odd looks. Even now I found that much of the time I'd go out with my tracheotomy exposed – an affectation which could be justified by those disabled lobbyists who believe the public should be exposed to the reality of disfigurement, but which I couldn't justify since letting air unfiltered by the trachy-cover into my lungs wasn't a good idea. Most of the time it was simply a case of forgetting and it wasn't until I'd notice a shopkeeper was talking to my neck that I'd realise that I was uncovered.

I could understand that most patients didn't try to think of their tumour as computer art or their mask as a decorative artefact, but I was surprised that not one of the thousands of patients Henk had dealt with wanted to confront their cancer physically.

In any other hospital, I am sure, I would have been given the standard flannel. It is not hospital policy... it's impossible to get them out of store... I've lost the key to the store-room. Henk simply said 'I'll see what I can do' and went off to make a phone call.

Five minutes later Nigella and I were in the bowels of the hospital in one of the histopathology labs overseen by Cyril Fisher. I'd forgotten how nostalgic a hospital lab would be, and how many childhood memories I had of being taken to meet Dad at one or other of labs he ran. There was the same warm-acrid smell, the same jumble of tubes and wires and warning messages scrawled in felt-tip pen, the same whirrings coming from centrifuge and microtome and stirrer. I'm sure this lab was a technological miracle compared to the ones in which Dad had worked, but it looked and felt and smelled just the same to me. And there was for just a moment the childhood-inspired feeling that if these people in their white coats were looking after my cancer then I was in safe hands. There are those for whom the white coat, the test-tube, the smell of formaldehyde represent the unknown and the terrifying: for me they still have a comforting homeliness.

Cyril Fisher was a chirpy man, smiling, shortish, lab-coated and, as far as I can tell, like everyone here, the best in his field. He sat below a series of lengthy shelves fat with bound editions of cancer journals stretching back for years and in front of him was a four-way microscope, which is to say one with four sets of eyepieces focused on a single slide. He seemed to think it entirely reasonable that I should want to see the excrescence which was trying to kill me. Or if not reasonable then not the whim of a mad fetishist.

Fisher had slides going all the way back to the original cyst and the biopsy performed at St George's which determined how

C

much more than a cyst it was. We each sat at a set of eyepieces and he slipped a slide under the lens. All I could see was a pink smudge. I tried adjusting the focus and eventually got a rather sharper version of the picture which had once been on my computer desktop. It was a sheet of lilac-stained tissue with a number of light circular markings. These were the benign cells, the cells which, left to their own devices, would get on with the job God or evolution had given them to do. Dotted around the place, though, were black dots: cancer cells. There were, as I'd been told at the time, very few of them and those that were there weren't clumped together in tumorous form.

But that was a slide from the cysts. Fisher found a section of the lump taken from my tongue: it was all cancer.

I don't know how I'd expected to feel at this confrontation – relief? anger? desolation? I was conscious of everyone in the room waiting for some sort of reaction from me, but I felt no difference between seeing my own cancer and seeing that of somebody else. It was out of me now: by that definition alone these weren't the killer cells even if there were some killer cells still around.

A couple of weeks later, and for the benefit of the cameras we went back, this time to have a look at the tumour proper. This did faze me slightly, and not because of its existence but because of its condition. Crowded together, the isolated cells of the first slide became a greyish lump of rubbery matter. Or, rather, a number of lumps of matter, because it had been carved out of my mouth slice by slice. This, I think, was the image I found difficult – of a man with his hand in my mouth, scraping bits off my tongue with a scalpel. Had Fisher presented me with a single golf ball of the stuff, removed as if in one go like a mouthful of melon scooped from the whole, I would have found it rather easier.

C

As we left the lab we came across the remains of the department's museum of jocular cancers: thick glass bottles full of formaldehyde in which were suspended cancerous testicles the size of small melons, organs horribly distended by their tumours, lone tumours, removed from their host organs. It was the last of my cancer fetishism: from here on in, I decided, I was going to be as wary of staring the truth in the face as all the other patients Henk had seen in his 25 years.

Except that buried under the fetishism was a genuine interest in what was happening to me, an interest aside from the emotional and practical problem of facing my own death. For it was at this time that I started really scaring myself.

As well as writing the column in *The Times*, I'd taken on another in the *Sunday Telegraph*. The *Telegraph* column appeared in that paper's *Rx* magazine which was devoted to those eternal Sunday subjects, health and fitness. My column was a Fleet Street first: my job each week was to rubbish one or other aspect of alternative medicine. Although the column attracted a ton of mail from those who thought it unfair that I be allowed to take my stand unchallenged by true believers in homoeopathy and reflexology and the rest, I was unperturbed. One of the reasons, after all, that I was keen to make my point was because of the number of papers and magazines running alternative medicine pages without ever the suggestion that these practices provided anything other than reasonable and proven remedies.

The column meant I had to get to know my enemy and I started hoarding books on both alternative and orthodox medicine. Both scared me.

Although few of the alternative books were about cancer specifically, many of them had chapters devoted to it. Almost invariably the prognoses they gave were gloomier than those

C

given in the populist mainstream books I'd been reading so far, and, as far as I could see, this was for two reasons.

The first is that although you can finish up in court for making unproved claims for any cure – which is why the adverts for ginseng and garlic tablets never speak in any but the most general terms – there are only two named diseases for which it's specifically illegal to claim an unsubstantiated cure; one is tuberculosis, the other cancer.

The second is that while alternative medicine can, for all sorts of reasons, be rather good at dealing with chronic and irritating conditions which are clinically defined and affect the quality of life without affecting life itself, it's lousy at dealing with diseases whose coming and going can be checked with blood test or microscope. Aside from straight bacterial and viral infections, the most common group of such diseases, and the one which induces the most anxiety, is cancer.

But if alternative medicine was up to any sort of job at all then it should be able to make some sort of dent in fatality statistics associated with cancer. Even so, whatever else the authors of the alternative handbooks claimed for their curative regimes, a cure for cancer was beyond almost all of them. Most of the books I came across made great claims about using, say, naturopathic remedies to hold cancer at bay and many of them suggested treatments for the individual symptoms of cancer. Many others, more usefully, proposed ways that cancer sufferers' quality of life might be improved as the length of that life shortened.

There were even some authors who argued that cancer wasn't cancer at all but an imbalance of this or a dissonance of that, and that only by readjusting these vital balances could a cure be wrought. The nearest any of the books came to claiming an all-out cure were those which recommended particular anti-cancer diets.

(I remain as sceptical of these diets as I do of most of the other remedies. My scepticism is tempered only slightly by a conversation I had with one of the radiographers. I was waiting my turn for zapping one day and mentioned the ludicrousness of one diet I'd been reading about. She agreed, and said that when she started at the hospital there used to be a nutter who, having refused radiotherapy on his own behalf, would come down and rail against those sitting in the radiotherapy waiting room, telling them they should abandon evil radiation and take up his magical diet.

'Criminal,' I said. 'You kicked him out, of course?'

'Well yes,' she said. 'We kicked him out regularly. The only thing was he did survive for years and the cancer did disappear.'

Which only goes to prove – well, nothing very much at all really, but I thought I'd pass it on in the name of fair dealing.)

So here we had all these regimes claiming the earth for their healing powers but unable to claim very much at all for their power against cancer. Meanwhile here was the medical orthodoxy claiming that over the decades it has made progress in treating certain cancers. It gives the angry alternativists a choice: either they can say that their practices work in some situations but not in others, such as cancer, or they can deny what appears to me to be the undeniable and say that in fact conventional medicine has made no more progress than alternative medicine. Some go further: they say that in fact it's the alternative practices which hold the secret of any available cure.

It's a personal thing, I realise, but I find it quite remarkable that anyone can publish a book which says avoid radiotherapy and shun the surgeon's knife; stick instead to the juice of the Bibbly Bobbly tree taken twice daily.

C

Having said all of which, it was those denying alternativists who would get me scared. What if they were right? What if the truth was that no life had ever been saved by radiotherapy and that there was every chance that my cancer would be made worse by being irradiated? What if the truth as pronounced by a couple of books was that the main effect of cancer surgery was to release stray cancer cells into the body, allowing them to set up home elsewhere?

What if the truth was that which I'd assumed to be the case from the start but which I'd been denying ever since I'd been given the 92 per cent chance of cure back in April: that cancer invariably did kill and that all we were arguing about was whether I'd be dead in six months or five years?

I turned to the medical books for solace, and got none. Those aimed at the general public were positive enough and if you read them very quickly through half-closed eyes you could bring yourself to believe that cancer was like pneumonia: pretty nasty while you had it, but unlikely to kill you in the long run.

It was the ones aimed at doctors, the ones which didn't feel the need to pull punches, that got me. While Rhŷs Evans had given me a two to one chance of a cure, a book baldly titled *Cancer and its Management*[2] told me that clear-up statistics on tongue cancer depended very much on where the tumour was discovered and that a tongue-tip cancer stood a much better chance of being licked than one like mine at the back of the tongue.

I would order the books over the Internet or sneak them from piles of review copies when I went into one or other of the papers I worked for, and carry them up to my room like a kid with

2. Second edn Robert Souhama and Jeffrey Tobias, Blackwell Science, 1997.

snaffled *Playboys*. I'd run through the indexes looking for the key words which would be attached, I knew, to the terrifying paragraphs: 'Tongue, cancer of the', 'radiotherapy', 'surgery', 'mortality'. And that night I would lie in bed certain that whatever treatment I was under would fail. I knew, for instance, that when Rhŷs Evans said he would have liked to have been able to cut a bit more healthy tissue from around the tumour in my tongue, what he meant was that he'd had to leave some possibly tumorous tissue in there. And I knew, as I lay wakeful in the dark, that the chances of the radiotherapy picking up *every* remaining cancerous cell were zero. I might be conned for a couple of years, but some day one of those cells would reappear at the centre of a new tumour in a new place.

This certainly wasn't the positive attitude that everyone was telling me was needed to get through the illness. But then again I didn't feel as if it were a negative attitude, either. The symptoms got me down from time to time – the honking voice and all the coughing and spluttering, the continual pain at the base of my throat, my inability to eat much more than the odd slice of solids to supplement my milky diet – but I seemed to be suffering rather less generalised existential angst than I did when long-term existence was a more promising prospect.

In any case, I'd come to the conclusion that whenever somebody told me how much good a positive attitude would do me, what they meant was how much easier a positive attitude would make it for them. Positivism meant we could all carry on as before, that they didn't have to think before they spoke and then get embarrassed about saying things that I hadn't even noticed bore some metaphorical relationship to what I was going through (not long before a woman had reddened and apologised almost on her knees for using the word cancer in the sentence 'I

C

think he was Leo but he may have been Cancer'). As long as I was positive it meant they didn't have to cope with the nasty thoughts.

As it happened, I suppose I was being positive. True, I would never be able to do that thing of grinning and shouting 'I'm fighting and I'm gonna *win*' because that wasn't really the relationship I had with the cancer. Nor could I pretend I didn't have the illness. On the other hand I wasn't whining too much, and I seemed to have subsumed the cancer into a day-to-day life which also included the day-to-day things which the non-cancerous enjoyed. With the manifest disease reduced to a loss of voice, a liquid diet and a painful throat, Nigella was probably suffering my cancer more than I was.

And then the cancer stopped.

Chapter 12

C

I say the cancer stopped: what I mean is that they stopped treating me for cancer. Whoopee? Not so as you'd notice, no.

The original, *EastEnder*-interrupting diagnosis had been passed on at the end of March; in April I'd started radiotherapy to the left side of my neck; at the end of June they'd started looking for the primary tumour; at the end of July I'd had the tumour removed; at its end they'd started radiotherapy on the right side of my neck and my tongue. Five months a cancer patient, cancer victim, cancer sufferer, cancer what have you.

And here we were in June sitting in Peter Rhŷs Evans' rooms again. He'd looked in my throat, felt around my tongue, stood behind me and examined my neck and chin and could find no sign of anything nasty. He'd grilled me on my current state of health: my weight was stable if not exactly climbing, the various pains were, we'd agreed some time ago, the result of surgery rather than of cancer, my voice was coming on, and I could waggle my attenuated tongue around in a way which suggested that the muscle tone might be returning.

In clinical terms, at least, I was cancer free and at the end of October Rhŷs Evans, who normally finished off each session by making a booking for the next week, said, 'Well, I don't think I need see you for a month.'

It was the sentence I'd been waiting to hear ever since I so pointedly didn't hear it after the first lot of radiation back in May. I should have whooped with delight. Instead I felt the first scratchings of panic. If Rhŷs Evans and the Marsden weren't going to look after me, who was?

In fact there was still the odd excuse to go back to the Fulham Road. There was the tracheostomy, for instance. I am not a squeamish man, and I'm sure I'd have been entirely capable of taking the pipe out of my throat, hosing it down and replacing it a couple of times a week, but I'd made a point of always looking somewhere else when one of the nurses suggested that this was what most trachy-owners did. In fact I'd never even seen the hole in my throat because the flange at the end of the tube covered it up. And so each Tuesday and Friday I'd sit in the room in Weston Ward and Mercel or Caroline or Fran or Gloria would pull out the old tube and put a new one in. In fact very soon afterwards the job would be given over to my local district nurse, a very un-Sister George-like woman called Liz who would scrub up in the kitchen a couple of times a week before sitting me down at the kitchen table, pulling out the tube and studying the trapped secretions for signs of what they might say about my throat or lungs.

But as long as I was seeing one Marsden person I had access to them all. Any dropped hint of remission, of pain, of something slightly dodgy would get me instant referral to the sanctuary of a Rhŷs Evans or a Breach or a Henk.

There was, for instance, Dr Williams' Pain Clinic.

Isn't that a wonderful title? Say it with me: Dr Williams' Pain Clinic. He has it on a little notice on his door – DR WILLIAMS PAIN CLINIC: PLEASE KNOCK – and one day I saw a scribbled sign on a wall: This Way To Dr Williams' Pain Clinic. I mentioned Dr Williams' Pain Clinic in *The Times* one week and got letters from all over the country asking for directions. It's understandable: in a certain mood the four words – Doctor, Williams, Pain, Clinic – contain everything the soul craves: succour, excitement, restitution and, um, Williams. I saw the proprietor of the pain clinic as stick-thin, madly grinning, tufts of straggly grey hair at the temples, a stained and misbuttoned waistcoat, and a wire connected to mains electricity in each hand. What I got was a slick young anaesthetist which, all things considered, was probably the better deal.

Rhŷs Evans had been suggesting I turn up at the pain clinic for weeks now, and had even booked me an appointment which I'd cancelled. I'm not sure why. Certainly I was in pain much of the time, and equally certainly the various patent mixtures of paracetamol and codeine weren't dealing with that pain. On the other hand I'd tried, however subconsciously, to avoid all those services which were too obviously for the terminal patients I would see hobbling about the hospital, blank-faced and patently in receipt of something intravenous and mind-numbing, and Dr Williams' Pain Clinic sounded just like that.

'It sounds like a dodgy German porn movie,' I said to Dr Williams when I eventually turned up. Unfortunately the sentiment demanded more of my post-operative elocutionary skills than I was able to give, and by the time I'd repeated it for the third time it had lost most of its edge.

'Yes,' said Dr Williams, catching on. 'I've tried to think of a different title, but nothing else works, you know?'

To say that Williams lived for pain is probably overstating the case, but as an anaesthetist he seemed to devote much of his time to relieving pain. Palliative care usually seems to be about letting people teeter towards the abyss in something like comfort, but Williams seemed as concerned with patients who would, or might, be cured but whose pain needed tending pending that cure.

The great thing about Williams was that he believed in aggressive pain relief with none of this mimsy be-brave-and-leave-it-for-as-long-as-possible-and-then-try-some-deep-breathing rubbish. Pills are what you need for pain: lots of pills. We went through Williams' repertoire of analgesia together. We talked about the various forms of mid-level relief like a couple of

C

Dutch hippies discussing brands of dope, and we worked out a way where I could take pain relief every hour or two without my kidneys packing up.

He tempted me with the morphine equivalent of a nicotine patch, and I said, 'Weellll... I don't know, how about I leave that one until I get better?' Again, this was a pride thing. Morphine was, as far as I was concerned, what you took when you had surrendered control to others and although, unlike the alternativists, I had no problem with this when it was necessary, I felt ambivalent about taking the drug as an advanced version of Disprin. At our first meeting I turned it down like a brave Scout; at the second I took home three boxes of the patches; at the third I complained it wasn't strong enough.

By the fourth, though, I'd stopped using it. In its patch form, Williams insisted, the risk of addiction was minimal but given that the standard analgesics seemed to be able to do the job I didn't see much reason for chancing my arm with a major opiate.

As it turned out Rhŷs Evans saw me before the month was up, in order to determine that it was time for the tracheotomy to come out. For the past couple of weeks I'd worn a red plastic button to close off the tracheotomy during the day and only opened the tube at night. The deal was that if I slept through the night twice with the button in place I'd be released from the tube. In fact I only made one and a half nights; on the second night I slept badly, took the button out for a minute and went back to sleep before remembering to replace it. It was enough, though: I was going to get my neck back.

More panic: the last time I'd breathed entirely through my own set of tubes I'd almost died. Even though I knew that most of the swelling which had caused my throat to close had gone down, I was worried. There was, said Rhŷs Evans, no need: the hole in my throat would take a while to close, during which time it would become apparent whether there would be any problems.

In fact the tube was taken out at midday and by 6 p.m. the hole, which had been some centimetre or more in diameter, had closed up; if I pinched my nostrils and closed my mouth I couldn't take a breath through my neck. That night I found myself dozing and waking as I had before the tube went in. The throat wasn't as swollen inside, but four months after the operation there was still enough oedema inside to match the one I could see dragging my chin down.

Sometimes the lack of oxygen caused me to jerk into wakefulness via oddly compact nightmares: tiny little single-act dreams with no plot line and just the one terrifying event to remind me that I was doing something dangerous. Like trying to breathe. After almost a week of more or less no sleep I broke into my Rhŷs fast again: he suggested an oxygen cylinder by the bed just to keep my levels up. It meant I got a few good nights' sleep and for a while stopped feeling like somebody the army are softening up for work as a grass in Belfast. The bad news was that while losing the tracheotomy was a major step towards looking like a normal person, and eventually talking and eating like one, sleeping with an oxygen tank beside the bed and a set of plastic cannulae connecting it to my nose was profoundly depressing. Only severely ill people sleep with oxygen at hand, or dying ones, and I liked to think that I was moving away from that estate.

But I never will.

True, there was that feeling of everything winding down. See me in the street and – unless I've not shaved for a couple of weeks, giving me half a beard on one side of my face but none on the other – you'd never know that a few months ago I was

C

strapped down with tubes while they decided where my cancer was. Most of the time I can make myself understood and I'm pretty sure that once the dark pain at the back of my throat has gone I'll be able to eat.

In theory, at least, and given a following wind, there's every chance that by the time this appears in the bookshops it will all be over. There will be the odd symptom there to remind me of what happened for most of '97: the voice will never be quite the same and, perfectly cut though they are, there will always be scars about my neck.

That could be true of dozens of illnesses and I have scars elsewhere on my body resulting from events I can't even remember. But the cancer scars are different. A broken leg is a broken leg, a case of pleurisy merely that. They are not predictors of broken legs or pleural infections yet to come. Even if I steel myself to imagine the best – that in five years I am still cancer free – I can't imagine that the virtual-viral form of cancer which infects the mind will be cured. In every possible way I will be reminded of what I was this year, and of what I will still be.

I can't imagine that even were I rather more well balanced than I am I will in two or ten or twenty years' time be able to run my tongue in its limited orbit round my mouth and feel an ordinary ulcer without my stomach clenching. Every sore throat from now on, however obviously connected to a cold or a night's drinking, will bring with it the possibility of cancer. How could it be otherwise? I have proved myself prone to cancer and, specifically, to cancer in and around the mouth. Having been let down by my treacherous immune system once, how can I ever trust it again?

What I don't know, is how that distrust will affect our life together, me and my body. Will it be like the relationship between the momentarily unfaithful husband accepted back into the home on condition of fidelity but with the crime always there as the ironic subtext to every conversation, argument, bout of love-making? Or will it simply replace the distrust I always had of my body, the certainty that it was never quite up to the job? Will I still have the fear of imminent death but not the panic attacks to go with it?

And if – when – it happens again will I have to go through the same mental processes for a second time or will the short cuts around my psyche which I've established this time hang around so that I can cut straight to the chase next time? My guess is that the first time you can accept the possibility of a cure and arrange your sense of terror to fit in with the medical optimism. A second time and you're there on your own.

Either way, it doesn't feel like a death sentence because I can only see it now in terms of the death sentence which hangs over all of us all of the time. Teenage suicides tend to be reductionist on this point: what is the point of living at all if all the time we are hurtling towards certain death? Religious fundamentalists take the same line with the caveat that the certain death is a good thing and the pointless life a test which precedes it. And rational people tend to be agnostics or religious in a lukewarm way because atheism or fundamentalism don't fudge those questions about our purpose which can only ever be fudged.

I fudge still and despite all, but what I now know is that thinking your reprieve from the death sentence has been cut from 78 or so years to 44 or so isn't the end I'd imagined it to be. For some reason, even in the lowest moments when I believed the doctors were stringing me along, when I could feel the travelling cancer gripping organs the precise location of which I wasn't quite sure ('Darling – where's the duodenum again?'), there were things to live for, to cram into the last years or months or days.

None of this, of course, is to say that it won't change. It may be that in a while, when I press the 'save as' button on the word processor and bundle these last thoughts off to the publisher (and that's 'last' as in 'get it all done in 70,000 words' rather than 'these be the last thoughts of the late John Diamond') I shall revert to the gibbering wreck I was, or slash my wrists or just one of them, or phone up the doctor and ask to go on to Valium for a year or two.

But meanwhile here I am on the page now in the present tense rather than the past. Slowly, slowly, things become dissociated from my cancer and become part of me. The week before last, for instance, I tripped over and broke – I thought – my big toe. I took it to casualty and for the first few minutes felt a certain proprietoriality about the place. At this time of the year with the medical school term just starting the chances are, after all, that I'd spent more time in hospitals than some of the housemen here. But gradually I relaxed. I wasn't a cancer patient with special rights, just another schlemiel who'd broken his toe.

It cuts both ways, though. Yesterday I opened the medicine cabinet and a large bottle of antioxidant vitamins (which I will surely start taking some day soon given their prophylactic action against cancer) dropped from a shelf and hit the wash-basin; the front half of the basin fell off and landed on my other big toe. I should, by rights, have taken the resultant cut to the hospital to be stitched. But I'd had enough of hospitals, I knew them too well. I dressed the wound myself, and rather well too, I thought.

Not long after Nigella and I started going out together in 1989 we found ourselves at one in the morning walking through Smithfield Market at the edge of the City. The market hadn't started up yet and the only real lights on in the area came from St Bartholomew's Hospital just across the road. We strolled over there, my arm around her shoulder, and into the hospital. I imagine that now we'd be stopped by some sort of security guard, but then we were free to wander around and confess to each other how secure we felt surrounded by the crazed tiles and the disinfectant smell and the signs pointing to the various medical sanctuaries.

Not now. Here is where I feel safe. I am sitting in my office at home. Nigella is out briefly, but will be back soon. On the floor below as I type I can hear Cosima shouting at the TV screen and Bruno giggling, and the sounds and smells are better than any hospital.

In an hour or so I will go down and make myself supper. Occasionally I force down a proper supper: half a plateful of steak pudding and peas, a third of a bowl of rice. There is the odd pear during the day, and the occasional surprise bowl of cereal. The amount of solid food I am taking has grown and will grow, I hope, further still. But because a small meal is still a mammoth task for me, I need my real calories and so tonight supper will be, as it has been most nights since they took the food tube away, a Scandishake diluted by half a pint of cream and topped up with half a bottle of liquid glucose. It will take 90 seconds to prepare and half that time to drink it, and when the last drop has left the glass I will spend half a minute trying to suck it into my throat and then another half-minute swilling the remainder out of my mouth with tap water and spitting the last mouthful into the sink. It's not pretty, but it's prettier than most of the alternatives.

If the drink hits my throat in just the wrong way then I shall break into a hacking cough which might last up to five minutes

C

and involve a lot more swilling and spitting, although if either of the children come into the kitchen I'll take my coughing into the bathroom.

Sometimes I worry about the children. Obviously I worry about them as potential semi-orphans (or fully so: there is rather more cancer in Nigella's family than in mine) but more often it's about whether cancer will still be around when they're my age and whether my grandchildren – known to me or otherwise – will look bemusedly on as their mother or father hacks post-operative mucus into the kitchen sink. Originally I'd intended somewhere in this book to make a punt at the future of cancer research, but I won't. I think I'd prefer to leave it up to the newspaper health correspondents who can talk only in terms of major breakthroughs, and the anti-science nutters who see evil in any possible cure.

In any case, the more I read about it the more I realise that the cure for cancer is as likely to come, if it comes at all, from some research fluke refined by unflukey science. There are times when I am sanguine, when I believe that if I can hold out for two or three years there will be new procedures around to keep me going for the next two or three. And there are times when I believe that all the research I've seen so far is based on the principle that when one door opens two more close and that great leaps in cancer-fighting science represent no more than tiny steps along a lengthy and convoluted path.

All of which leaves me – well, where?

I am still on the books of the Marsden as a cancer patient and shall be for years to come although there is no sign of cancer in me as far as anyone is aware, and even if it's my hunch that the cancer will return and probably sooner rather than later.

I have learned a lot about myself in nine months, and a lot

about those around me. Much of that knowledge is useful, liberating even. Equally much of it is banal stuff which I should have known anyway had I bothered to think about it. But the bad has outweighed the good a millionfold. While I have spent the bad times in bed with a book, Nigella has spent them running the house and the children and worrying about a sick husband. The children have passed through nine of their most formative months watching their father get progressively thinner, coughing his guts up, woozy from painkillers, scarred, tired, irritable.

It shouldn't be like this. That I can face the fact that it is like this is, I suppose, something. But what a bloody meagre something it is.

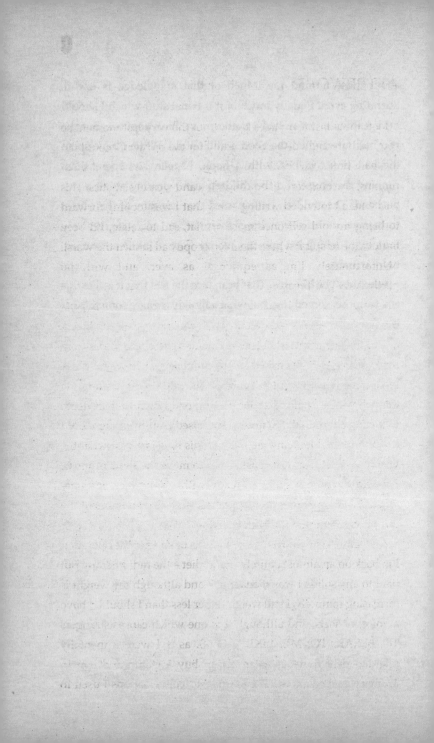

AFTERWORD

I'd left these last few pages blank until the very last moment so that, with the bulk of the book ready for the printers, I could nip in to sign off with a solid prognosis, a line to draw under the months, and chapters, of equivocation and weasel statistics. This was where I intended writing either that I was looking forward to being my old self once more or that, sad to relate, I'd been back to the hospital where the microscope had shown the worst.

Unfortunately I'm as equivocal as ever, and with no particularly good reason.

It is, as I write this, almost a year to the day since Nigella interrupted *EastEnders* to tell me I had cancer. Last week, during one of those particularly bleak moments I still come across from time to time, Nigella asked me to promise that however bleak the moments got I wouldn't commit suicide. On the assumption that we weren't talking about picking one's own time of death following a terminal diagnosis, I promised readily enough. But I don't think that had anyone told me this time last year what the year ahead held, and then asked me to make the same promise, I would have been quite so ready with reassurance. It's only when taken operation by operation and disappointment by disappointment that it's been bearable.

How am I? Who knows? Nine months or so after the operation I'm back on an almost entirely liquid diet – the radiotherapy put paid to any solids I was managing – and although my weight is increasing minutely, I still weigh rather less than I should. I have a voice, of sorts, and although it is one which causes strangers TO. SPEAK. TO. ME. LIKE. T-H-I-S. as if I were a mentally retarded deaf mute, it means I can buy a stamp and join in ordinary conversations. The journalists' conversations I used to

C

like so much – where the trick was to say as much as possible before the next person – are still beyond me. I'll leap in with some gabbled *bon mot* and the badinage will crash to a halt while I repeat slowly something which usually doesn't bear repetition. Although I still have to talk with a handkerchief at the ready and there are days when I have to write things down for shopkeepers because I can't be bothered repeating them, everyone tells me that my voice is coming on apace. Last week I even started using the phone again.

As for broadcasting, it turns out that although the medical experts were gaily telling me there was every chance of my getting back in front of a microphone last November, nobody much expected me to be able to wield a microphone in time for last year's contracted shows. Their optimism was to encourage my own: they thought it would be useful for me to have something to aim for.

The other week, concerned, they took a series of biopsies from my mouth: to our joint relief, all turned out to be clear. I see Peter Rhŷs Evans once a month and I haven't seen Michael Henk or been into the Marsden for two or three months now. When people ask me if I still have cancer, and they do, I feel as if I ought to say that I haven't because the truth is that there is no cancer anyone can find. But when it comes to saying the words, I can't do it. I hedge, and fudge, and bluster. 'Who knows?' I say, and 'Ask me again in five years.'

I still feel ill. In part it's the obvious physical deformities – the scars and the talking problems. I'm also in pain for much of the time. I still wear a morphine patch and take handfuls of painkillers to deal with the pain in my throat and its associated earache, and my tongue and oedemic neck and chin are still sore. I have to sleep upright because with my saliva glands gone I still have mucus problems. I have no real sense of taste and retain a propensity for long coughing jags that keep me out of cinemas and the theatre.

But most worrying of all is the tiredness. Nobody has told me to worry about tiredness, but I know it to be a symptom of recurrent cancer. True, I'm getting almost no sleep and I suppose that even now I'm getting over the operation and the subsequent radiotherapy. But there are times when waves of extreme torpor overcome me such that I nod off at the strangest times including, to my distress, while I was waiting for the lights to change the other day.

In short I'm by no means convinced that the worst is over.

But for all that I'm happy enough most of the time. I've been offered both drugs and counselling to deal with the sadness and anger I still feel from time to time, but after some purely nominal thought I've turned both down. After all, it's not as if anger and depression aren't perfectly valid responses to what's been going on. My family is wonderful and, fearful that I might not be with the kids as long as I'd intended, I spend rather more time with them than I have been recently. Long-suffering Nigella has taken to disappearing with them for long periods at weekends so that I could rest but thankful as I was at the time I now rather regret that missed time and I'd prefer to be tired with them than rested without. I've also been writing more than ever before. There was a brief period when some of that extra writing was concerned with the debate which briefly took over the media columns of the press about whether columnists should write about their cancer, but most of my extra writing has had nothing to do with cancer at all.

A couple of nights ago I was sitting with Nigella in bed.

'What are you smiling at?' she said.

C

I didn't realise that I was, but what I was thinking about was Nigella and the children. I was holding a soft toy which Bruno had brought into the bed when Cosima had fetched him in that morning.

'It's such a strange time, isn't it?' I said.

'How so strange?'

'Oh you know. Strange in that I've never felt more love for you than I have in the past year, that I've never appreciated you as much, nor the children. In a way I feel guilty that it should have taken this to do it, I suppose. But it is strange, isn't it.'

For the first time, I found myself talking like this without resenting that it had taken the cancer to teach me the basics, without resenting that there was part of me capable of talking like a 50s women's magazine article without blushing.

I still don't believe that there is any sense in which the cancer has been a good thing but, well, it is strange, isn't it?

THE LAST WORD

Just after David Bowie started appearing on stage with that ludicrous early-70s haircut, or Boy George posed for the first of a thousand over-made-up publicity stills, or any punk did any of the affectedly spontaneous things that punks were wont to do during that sour period of British pop, they all confessed much the same thing to any passing journalist who'd stop to listen. They didn't understand, they said, what all the fuss was about. After all, they had been walking round the playground of (insert local high school) dressed like this for years now because that was the sort of individualistic, go-my-own-way guys they were. And if the media wanted to make something of the haircut or the makeup or the dried-on vomit, well that was up to the media.

Oh yeah, I used to think. So why was it that we never saw any of these Boy George manques queuing up for school dinners in their turquoise eye shadow and Boots No 7 blusher? Why did we never see any of the Boy Toms and Bill Zowies who didn't make it to the top but were, nonetheless, doing their own thing in playgrounds round the country? There was, we knew, a bandwagon, and they were jumpers-on it.

Except that this is now the position I find myself in.

When I started writing about my cancer it was as a columnist in a national newspaper. When I say I had no idea how long I'd be writing about it for that's just what I mean. It was entirely possible that my editor at *The Times* might have restricted my mentioning the cancer to once a month on grounds of taste or circulation. It seemed at the time (but not now: boy, not now) that this might be something seen off with six weeks of radiotherapy and thus make too small a wave in my personal pond to rate much of a mention on the page. Conversely it might have been that I only had six weeks of writing left in me, for although it seemed apparent that whatever the eventual outcome I would live for at least another year or so, there was no saying what sort of writing I'd be capable of at any point along that line.

By the time this book first appeared in hardback, things had changed. I'd written 40 or 50 columns about my illness, made a film for the BBC about it, turned up on any number of TV and radio shows to promote the book and the film. Journalists who specialised in writing while their lower lip trembled came round and wrote pieces in the tabloid press about my pale fragility or, as the whim took them, my dark inner strength.

Meanwhile something had developed which was described by those in the business of describing such things as 'the confessional writing industry'. Ruth Picardie had, as I noted in the book, written about her own terminal cancer and there were at least three books on the shelves aside from mine from media-industry cancer patients. The result was any number of articles in the national press asking where cancer sufferers got off describing their condition on the printed page and others suggesting that whatever we wrote couldn't be the whole truth which must be too terrifying to confine to print. I turned up on television a couple of times to shout at people who insisted that writing about illness was a new trend and Nigella went on the radio to look scornfully in the direction of a poor journalistic sap who'd been double-dared by her magazine editor into writing something nasty about the cancer patients.

It was, I suppose, as grist to the mill, but each word of the 'confessional industry' description offended. 'Industry' suggested smoking chimneys with identical products plopping off the end of a line, 'confessional' that in writing about my cancer I was admitting to something of which I should be ashamed.

More: the complaint made journalistic nonsense. If I'd gone to my editor and said that I'd learned that cancer affected a third of the population and might soon affect half of it, and that on this basis I wanted to find your typical cancer patient and report on his progress over the year, nobody would have regarded it as other than a long-term newspaper series. Certainly nobody would have suggested that it was impossible for a journalist to get at the truth of such an emotionally charged story and thus that he should leave it alone altogether? After all, journalists write about such emotionally charged subjects as rape and murder all the time and nobody suggests these lie. But because the subject of my progress report was me it counted not as reporting but as confession.

But as I complained about this traducement of my writing I knew I sounded just like the boy who had cut his hair en brosse on top, left it long at the back, drawn a zig-zag across his gaunt face and was claiming to have been a Spider from Mars since junior school. It was true: there were a lot of us about the place suddenly.

And I have to admit that realisation altered the way I wrote for a while. I started writing apologetic pieces which had as their subtext the supposition that the readers must be bored with the story by now, glib tracts which relied on a sort of 'Take my oncologist – I wouldn't say he was fat but . . .', vaudeville patter.

But then the illness itself altered and I found myself writing something like the truth again.

By July 1998 I was putting on weight, albeit by downing three drinks each day which Nigella would concoct to be as calorific as possible. I was still unable to eat solids for the simple reason that

C

as long as my tongue was effectively atrophied I had no way to get the food to the back of my mouth and into my throat. But still I thought – or pretended I thought – that I continued on the road to recovery. I would turn up at the speech therapist's once a week and go through my exercises, and occasionally I'd make some minor breakthrough – a phone conversation which didn't require too many repetitions or a party conversation where a joke got a laugh.

But somehow I never really believed it.

I'd started developing some new pains in my mouth. Most of these were fly-by-night twinges, remnants of the old hypochondria, but one of them stayed with me and was obviously something substantial. Whenever I drank anything I would get the sharpest pain at the back of what remained of my tongue. Nigella and I took the pain off to Peter Rhŷs Evans for inspection and eventually he reported that it was a sinus which was trapping liquid. The first time he told us this, the sinus was a benign thing, an accidental cul-de-sac which had formed in among the scar tissue, but gradually over the next couple of weeks it became something more intrusive. It was, of course, the cancer returning. Or, as likely, it was the cancer-never-gone and that the margin of safety of the removed tumour had, as had been hinted, been too small for safety after all.

Before the operation in 1997 I'd been handed the standard it's-not-our-fault-guv disclaimer to sign on which was detailed the nature of the procedure I was to undergo. I wrote in above the description the rider that however bad the tumour appeared to be they should not perform a total glossectomy – which is to say remove the whole of my tongue. Looking back on it now this seems a futile sort of gesture. If the only cure was removing my whole tongue then what point was there leaving it there? I wrote at the time that there would have been serious competition between living without a tongue and dying with one, but looking back now, I'm not so sure. Then again, at the time I still had no idea how long this road could run or how far down it I was prepared to go.

Preparing for the big operation I assumed that this was as much as a man could take and that on top of the crippled voice, the radiotherapy, the radical diet, this would be the worst. The truth is that when I inserted that rider it wasn't because I didn't want them to remove the tongue but that I couldn't conceive of a state of tonguelessness and that denying it on the consent form was my acknowledgement of that.

Now here we were again in Rhŷs Evans' Harley Street rooms listening to details of the next operation which was, of course, to remove the rest of my tongue.

When I wrote in Chapter 9 about the original operation I pointed out that the waggly little thing we refer to as the tongue is only that organ's visible tip. On the plastic cut-away model of the face and throat on Rhŷs Evans' desk, the dull pink tongue descended way into the back of the throat and, at the front, down into the lower jaw, filling the space of the chin. This time plastic surgery would be needed: a lump of muscle in my back would be cut out and used to replace the tongue. For a while I thought this meant the recreation of a new tongue, of something which would have some of the function of the old one. But no: the flap would be no more than a platform, filling in the empty space in my lower jaw.

Worse: along with the tongue the surgical team would be relieving me of my epiglottis (the flap which stops food and drink going down the wrong way) and the mass of sub-lingual folds above the vocal chords. It meant that the only protection I

C

had against food and drink descending into my lungs would be my vocal chords; organs not really prepared for that job. It meant that while I may one day be able to learn to take minimal sustenance through my mouth, the chances are that I'd do most of my eating from the day of the operation through a tube they'd insert into my stomach.

The conversation with Rhŷs Evans was an odd one. It reminded me of the sorts of conversation I used to have with teachers after I'd received a D for a test paper for which I was blithely expecting an A and in which they pointed out that academic traits which I'd always assumed they rather liked were in fact proving the educational death of me. Rhŷs Evans spoke of those symptoms which he'd suspected all along might lead to this moment, but they were symptoms which until now I thought indicated recovery. I'd thought I was getting some movement back into my tongue and indeed every time he'd inspected it he'd refer to this developing skill approvingly. But now it seemed that this was nowhere near the movement one would expect of a recovering tongue and to his expert eye showed that the blood wasn't getting to the tongue properly. There was the pain which, until now, we'd always discussed as a by-product of the operation rather than of the cancer; now I learned that this was just what cancer pain felt like.

The only slightly optimistic note came from Rhŷs Evans' suggestion that the effect on my voice might not be too bad, and that with luck and given the poor recovery of my tongue, I might eventually be able to speak as well without a tongue as I was currently doing with three-quarters of one. Optimistic as this briefly sounded, it meant, apart from anything else, that I'd never broadcast again. In fact I'd done quite a bit of radio in the past couple of months: I'd had a piece in the last edition of

Fourth Column and did a dozen or so radio interviews and a couple of TV programmes to promote the hardback edition of the book. But all of them were done as a man with a dodgy voice: there was never any suggestion that I could appear on radio or TV except as a man talking about the problems of his corrupted voice.

We all sat quietly for a few moments while I took in the offer of this new operation. I couldn't think properly. This was worse, somehow, than even the original diagnosis. I felt the oppressive weight of the interminable surgical process suddenly, slicing me inch-by-inch, suckering me into ever more drastic remedies, ever more unbearable disabilities.

'What happens', I said, 'if I don't have the operation?' Rhŷs Evans described the slow growth of the tumour as it descended towards my larynx, stopping me speaking and eventually stopping me breathing.

Nigella and I walked out into Harley Street reeling, and sat in the car.

When I was 11 I got a Hackney scholarship to the City of London school. I'd been a bright child in junior school and used to being at the top of the class without working very hard for it. At the City of London I was in a class full of bright children and, worse, bright children who worked hard. At the end of the first year I came near the bottom of the class, a position I had no resources to deal with. As I travelled home with my school report I tried to work out something to say to my parents which would take the shock of my failure away in an instant, something which would cancel it out. I got home, knocked on the door and when mum answered it I said, without preamble 'I want to leave the school. It's not right for me.' Somehow – wrongly - I imagined that my parents would take me at my word

C

and ignore the damning report as symptomatic of the school's failure rather than mine.

I felt the same sort of blind panic now. Sitting in the car I needed a quick and radical solution to this: a solution to the prognosis, the threat of the surgery, the prospect of the tongueless, voiceless, foodless life. I told Nigella I was seriously thinking of not having the operation. And then seizing on the quick solution I asked her if she'd help me commit suicide. She wouldn't – not because, as the complete athiest, she had any moral argument with suicide itself, but for a list of other reasons which included wanting me to hang around as long as possible and not wanting to have to tell the children one day when they asked that she'd helped the father they couldn't remember kill himself.

The thought went away for a while; we drove home.

I had the operation a couple of days later in August '98. This time there was no question of my not accepting all the help I could get and I started on antidepressants a couple of days before the operation in the hope that they'd kick in just as the morphine was wearing off. The routine was much the same as it had been the last time: a few days in the High Dependency Unit, a few more days with tubes poking from me back in my room. This time I seemed more able to cope with the hospital routine and lasted in hospital for the full fortnight so that when I came home I was relatively normal, as far as the children were concerned, always remembering that these were children who were getting used to their father's cumulative disablement.

I had a tracheotomy again and now I had a tube poking out of my stomach through which I would feed three times a day. I brought home two carrier bags full of drugs, sprays, wipes, swabs and so on, and a schedule for taking the various pain killers, anti-emetics, food supplements, indigestion remedies and so on which would cover me for the next few weeks. I also wore a small battery-operated pump which would inject a regular flow of dimorphine into me to keep the pain down. I had scars at the left-hand side of my neck where they reached through to get the tongue, and for about a foot along my back where they'd taken the muscle and its attached vein. Looking at myself in the mirror I realised that if I'd had all three operations at the same time my head would have fallen off: I now had a series of scars almost entirely encircling my neck.

I had no voice to speak of because my new tongue was still bloated and full of stitches, but within weeks it became apparent that while Nigella and the children could understand almost everything I said, nobody else was ever likely to be able to.

But strangely I felt convinced that the worst was over and that I was cancer-free. I also felt deeply depressed. I would lie in bed calculating how best to do away with myself. I knew, for instance, that I had a bottle of sleeping pills somewhere which I could crush up and pump into my stomach: one afternoon I went as far as to count them and look up lethal dosages in one of my medical books. It seemed, in those days, such a reasonable thing to do – to let it all just slip away from me. Indeed it's possible that the only reason I didn't do it then was because I'd promised Nigella that if I was going to digress from the stated regime I'd consult with her first, and I knew the reasons she'd have for not killing myself were reasonable ones.

And so here I was: my tongue gone, unable to speak or eat and no real chance of doing either for as long as I lived. It wasn't quite as miserable as it sounds. The antidepressant started to do its job and I started to have a shot at living a little. In September, for instance, Nigella held a party to launch her first book which

C

was, ironically enough, about food. I'd intended turning up briefly, smiling a forced smile, and slipping away, but I found myself the last to leave. In part it was because I was so proud of Nigella's success, and in part because I was having a genuinely good time. It turned out that I could be almost as jokey with a pad and pencil as I was with my old voice, and even better, I was able to drink again. I'd hardly touched a drop recently because of the soreness of my mouth and throat, but here I was pumping the stuff into my stomach tube with a large plastic syringe, and far from finding it gross, friends lined up to watch. The Maître d' of the swish hotel bar in which the party was held even went so far as to show me how to get champagne into the syringe without filling it full of bubbles.

And so it went until the end of the year. Sure, there was the odd problem with the hole in my neck which was strangely unwilling to heal, and the voice I had seemed to be raspier than usual, but there were some wonderfully good times with the children and Nigella during which, tongue or no, I'd never felt happier. In December Peter Rhŷs Evans took one of his regular looks down my throat and pronounced himself mystified by the un-healed hole. Would I, he asked, pop in for a scan sometime? We fixed the date for sometime in the New Year and both Nigella and I pretended that we believed this was a routine event when both of us knew it might well not be. On this basis we decided that we should take the kids away for a holiday: we hadn't had one for two years or more and if I needed even more surgery then this would be our only opportunity for a while.

We spent the end of 1998 and the start of 1999 in Disney World and had a wonderful time. Transporting a week's worth of liquid food took some doing and there were a couple of days when I stayed in bed, knackered, while Nigella and the kids went off to the Magic Kingdom, but that and my inability to do the junk food which is so much a part of theme park life aside, we could hardly have enjoyed it more.

A couple of days after we returned I went for the scan. There was, indeed, some suggestion of returning cancer around my larynx. If a biopsy proved this to be the case then we were, apparently, talking about a total laryngectomy. My voice box would be removed as the surgeons chased the cancer down my gullet and the result would be almost no voice at all, a tracheostomy for life but – the upside – the possibility that I might be able to swallow liquids again.

I went in for the biopsy and the next day turned up for the results. I'd prepared my *Times* readers for a week or so off while I had the operation I was sure I'd need. In the event I did write a column the next week:

I know what I said last week and that I wasn't meant to be here today: as we speak I should be back on the ward with the surgeons chasing the cancer further down my neck. But as soon as we arrived at the outpatients clinic we knew it was all up. Normally, and despite BUPA's hefty chequebook, we conduct our clinical meetings in an ordinary white cubicle in the general outpatient's clinic; this time the receptionist gave us a tight smile and said Mr Rhŷs Evans had asked for us to be shown over to one of the chain-hotel designed consulting rooms in the Marsden's private wing. You do not ask for your patients to be taken to the comfy chairs if you're about to tell them that after all the shadow on the scan was a packet of Woodbines left on the machine by one of the cleaners.

When Rhŷs Evans arrived it was with the unspoken hint of worse news still. The list of clinical possibilities thus far have all

C

been either surgical or radiological and I've known for some time that if a medical doctor ever turned up to a consultation then we were no longer talking about cure but about remission. Accompanying my surgeon were two men I'd not met before: a consultant medical oncologist and his registrar. Standing behind them, looking embarrassed, was a tallish man in hood and gown with a scythe over his shoulder.

Statistics tell us that anyone whose job is treating those diagnosed as having cancer will, in around 60% of cases, eventually have to dole out the worst possible news, and you'd suppose that after some years of doing it most doctors would find a way somewhere between the mawkish and the unnecessarily brusque which would serve them comfortably in the majority of cases. I suppose it's testimony to Peter Rhŷs Evans that he gave us the news white-faced, nervous, with eyes downcast, much as he must have given the news the first time he ever had to, as if it were something both unsayable and already said.

And the news is this:

The cancer is in too many places around my throat and neck to warrant any more surgery. I could ask for a second opinion, I suppose, but quite honestly it's bad enough having one expert telling you how soon you're going to die without bringing in a second to rub it in. If I leave the cancer to take its natural course I have about six months left. If I have chemotherapy, and assuming the chemotherapy works in my case and that it's not so arduous as to be unbearable, then I might double or treble that time and there's a small but significant chance of my doing even better than that given that the cancers are tiny and I feel healthier than I ever have.

I'll take the chemotherapy, of course. Why would I not?

I'd imagined that I'd feel terrified when I got the news, but what I felt most of all was sad. Sad for Nigella, for the children, for my parents. As if, of course, sad were a word up to this particular job. I realised that the reason I don't seem to be going through the standard denial-anger-bargaining with God-acceptance schtick is because that's what I've been doing for the past 20 months or so. As soon as I heard the first diagnosis I heard a death sentence being passed and I suppose I never thought of the various operations and procedures as much more than temporary reprieves. Living with cancer must always mean living with the threat of death even, I imagine, if you manage to increase the distance between you and the diagnosis to the five years which counts as a cure.

Meanwhile I have some affairs to get in what passes for order. We haven't told the children yet and won't for a while at least and so if you come across them – and some of you, I know, do – please don't say anything. I'll carry on working for as long as I can and given that one of the side-effects of the chemotherapy is fatigue, I'm sure you'll understand if I don't answer all your mail individually from now on. And we're planning a big party for March to celebrate Nigella and my ten years of being together. Its strange, isn't it, how in the middle of all this madness there are some things worth celebrating?

And so this is how you find me. Not quite waiting to die, because although I've accepted that I will, and sooner rather than later, the same rules apply to the foreshortened life as to the one of normal length: just as no well-balanced 45 year old says 'Why bother going to the movies? I'll be dead in 30 years' so I find that my imminent death doesn't stop me wanting to know what happens at the end of bad detective thrillers or wanting to

C

spend time with Nigella and the children. Those things are still worth doing.

As I write this we have all just returned from buying a basket for the spaniel we are due to collect in a couple of days time. A friend e-mailed me when she heard this to tell me about how it's a denial of what's happening and what's about to happen. It isn't at all: I know what's happening. But a dog is a happy thing, and it will be happy for me for whatever time I've got left and as happy as things can be for the family when I've gone.

London, March 1999